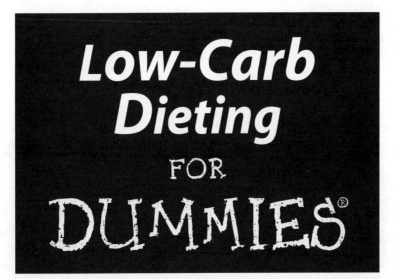

Low-Carb Dieting FOR DUMMIES®

by Katherine B. Chauncey, PhD, RD

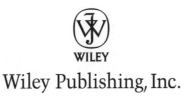

WILEY

Wiley Publishing, Inc.

Low-Carb Dieting For Dummies®
Published by
Wiley Publishing, Inc.
111 River Street
Hoboken, NJ 07030-5774
www.wiley.com

Low-Carb Dieting For Dummies®

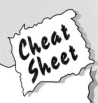

How to Eat Smarter

✔ Build your meals around fruits, vegetables, and lean protein food sources.

✔ Choose whole grains or legumes for your daily carb choices. Minimize your intake of processed foods.

✔ Choose very-low-fat milk and dairy foods.

✔ Choose monounsaturated rather than saturated fats.

✔ Eat three or four meals per day. Never starve yourself and never skip meals. If you eat between meals, eat Green Light foods, such as apples or oranges for a healthy, filling snack.

✔ Do not eat a full meal right before bedtime. A bedtime snack such as nonfat yogurt or cottage cheese and fruit is okay.

✔ Drink plenty of water — eight glasses a day.

✔ Exercise moderately 30 to 60 minutes at least five times a week.

✔ Practice the 90-percent/10-percent rule: Follow this plan 90 percent of the time, and treat yourself to a favorite food 10 percent of the time.

How to Stick with the Plan

✔ **Set up your kitchen for success.** Always have low-carb-friendly foods on hand ready to eat. Remove as many irresistible temptations as possible.

✔ **Avoid excessive hunger.** Eat before you're starving. When you're ravenous, making a healthy choice is tougher.

✔ **Prepare snacks in grab-and-go sizes.** Make prepackaged snacks from cut-up veggies and whole-wheat crackers in resealable plastic bags. Fresh fruit is already prepackaged for your convenience, so carry some wherever you go.

✔ **Eat a variety of foods.** Make sure you eat a variety of foods for better nutrition.

✔ **Find activities and exercises that you enjoy.** If you find something you really enjoy, you're more apt to do it every day. If you're social, find friends to walk with. If you look forward to exercise as your "alone time," plan times when you can work out alone. Make your workout personal.

✔ **Forgive yourself when you fail.** Everyone experiences a setback from time to time. Don't use it as an excuse to give up completely. Figure out where you went wrong and get going again!

How to Evaluate Portion Sizes

To determine the number of servings you're eating, you need to estimate portion sizes. You'll be surprised to see that normal portion sizes are a lot smaller than you think. Here are some hints:

Measurement	Size	Measurement	Size
½ cup	About the size of a cupcake wrapper	1 ounce cheese	About the size of your thumb or a pair of dice
1 cup	About the size of a tight fist or a tennis ball	3 ounces meat	About the size of the palm of a woman's hand or a deck of cards
1 medium fruit	About the size of a tight fist or tennis ball	2 tablespoons reduced-fat salad dressing	About the size of a Ping Pong ball
1 medium potato	About the size of a computer mouse	1 teaspoon oil or butter	About the size of the tip of a thumb

Low-Carb Dieting For Dummies®

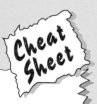

Green-Light Snack List

Here's a quick list of snacks to keep you going. Enjoy these snacks anytime, as often as you like. For more Green-Light suggestions, take a gander at Chapter 5.

- A juicy orange, an apple, a bunch of grapes, a handful of raisins, dried apricots
- An 8-ounce container of low-fat yogurt
- A can of unsweetened applesauce, diced peaches, or mixed fruit
- A glass of skim, ½%, or 1% milk
- Raw vegetables with low-fat salad dressing
- Sliced turkey rolled up in a lettuce leaf
- Boiled shrimp with zesty cocktail sauce
- Skim-milk mozzarella string cheese

Must-Haves for the Low-Carb Pantry

- Canned or bottled foods:
  - Tuna, salmon, or sardines (in water)
  - Vegetables (asparagus, carrots, green beans, mushrooms, and so on)
  - Fruit packed in light syrup or juice
  - 100-percent fruit preserves
  - Chicken or beef bouillon
  - Canned tomatoes and tomato paste
  - Salsa or ketchup
  - Canned or dried beans such as pinto, navy, kidney, lima, garbanzo, peas
  - Fat-free refried beans
  - Natural or low-sugar peanut butter
  - Sun-dried tomatoes
  - Artichoke hearts
  - Olives
  - Capers
  - Marinated vegetables (okra, beans)
  - Roasted peppers
  - Pickles and pickle relish
  - Horseradish, Dijon, spicy, or plain mustard
  - Red and white table wine (for cooking)
- Grains:
  - Whole-grain pasta, long-grain rice, wild rice, flours, and cornmeal
  - Oatmeal
  - High-fiber, no-sugar cereals
  - Low-sugar granola or homemade granola
  - Quinoa
  - Roasted soynuts
- Seasonings:
  - Salt-free seasonings
  - Garlic and onion, minced and powder
  - Bouillon cubes or sprinkles
  - Reduced-sodium soy sauce or Worcestershire sauce
  - Sugar substitutes
- Oils and vinegars:
  - Nonstick vegetable oil spray
  - Healthy oils (olive oil, canola oil, peanut oil, or light combination oils)

For Dummies: Bestselling Book Series for Beginners

About the Author

Katherine Chauncey, PhD, RD, is an Associate Professor in the Department of Family and Community Medicine at Texas Tech University School of Medicine. She is actively involved in medical student and resident education. She received her BS from the University of Arkansas and her MS and PhD from Texas Tech University. Dr. Chauncey is a licensed registered dietitian and a certified diabetes educator. She has over 25 years of experience in the field of nutrition.

Dr. Chauncey maintains a clinical nutrition practice and participates in patient care activities within the School of Medicine. She works with all age groups providing medical nutrition therapy for chronic illness. Her research interests focus on medical student and resident education and clinical nutrition interventions for diabetes, metabolic syndrome, and obesity.

Dr. Chauncey is a Fellow of the American Dietetic Association and member of the Society of Teachers of Family Medicine. She is a frequent speaker to professional and public groups.

Dedication

To those who are looking for a healthier way to do low-carb.

Author's Acknowledgments

I want to extend a sincere thanks to the hard-working team at Wiley Publishing. A special thanks to Pam Mourouzis for starting me in the right direction, and to Norm Crampton, Acquisitions Editor, for continuing the process. Norm's insight and good humor were always motivating. I appreciate Project Editor Elizabeth Kuball for her attention to detail and for keeping the project on track. I wish to thank Emily Nolan for her careful testing of all the recipes and Patty Santelli for her nutritional analysis.

A very special thank you goes to Heather Dismore for her creative and intelligent ideas. Her invaluable assistance made the writing of this book fun and enjoyable.

I am very grateful to my friend and colleague, Kathy Kolasa, PhD, RD, for her careful technical review of the book.

Thanks to my agent, Grace Freedson, for her warm support and guidance.

A big thank-you goes to Marilyn Beavers, Carol Chauncey, Jim Chauncey, Mildred Chauncey, Betty Kendrick, Sharon Mandrell, and Harold and Bertie Jo Priddy for allowing their great recipes to be included in this book.

And, of course, last but definitely not least, I am grateful to my husband, Jim, and my son, Matt. They are constant sources of joy and encouragement in my life. A special thanks to Jim, for his patience and encouragement during the writing of this book and to our son, Matt, for encouraging me since he was a child with, "Mom, you should write a book."

Publisher's Acknowledgments

We're proud of this book; please send us your comments through our Dummies online registration form located at www.dummies.com/register/.

Some of the people who helped bring this book to market include the following:

Acquisitions, Editorial, and Media Development

Project Editor: Elizabeth Kuball

Acquisitions Editor: Norm Crampton

Technical Editor: Kathryn Kolasa, PhD, RD

Recipe Tester: Emily Nolan

Nutrition Analyst: Patty Santelli

Senior Permissions Editor: Carmen Krikorian

Editorial Manager: Michelle Hacker

Editorial Assistant: Elizabeth Rea

Cover Photo: © Jeff Zaruba Studio/CORBIS

Cartoons: Rich Tennant, www.the5thwave.com

Production

Project Coordinator: Erin Smith

Layout and Graphics: Seth Conley, Stephanie D. Jumper, Heather Ryan, Brent Savage, Jacque Schneider, Shae Wilson, Erin Zeltner

Illustrator: Elizabeth Kurtzman

Proofreaders: Laura L. Bowman, Andy Hollandbeck

Indexer: TECHBOOKS Production Services

Publishing and Editorial for Consumer Dummies

Diane Graves Steele, Vice President and Publisher, Consumer Dummies

Joyce Pepple, Acquisitions Director, Consumer Dummies

Kristin A. Cocks, Product Development Director, Consumer Dummies

Michael Spring, Vice President and Publisher, Travel

Brice Gosnell, Associate Publisher, Travel

Kelly Regan, Editorial Director, Travel

Publishing for Technology Dummies

Andy Cummings, Vice President and Publisher, Dummies Technology/General User

Composition Services

Gerry Fahey, Vice President of Production Services

Debbie Stailey, Director of Composition Services

Contents at a Glance

Recipes at a Glance

· ·

Appetizers and Snacks

Beverages

Desserts

Entrees

Salads and Dressings

Side Dishes

Soups

Table of Contents

Introduction

. . . .

*W*elcome to *Low-Carb Dieting For Dummies.* You've probably heard a lot in the media, as well as from friends and family, about the benefits of low-carb dieting. That may be what encouraged you to pick up this book and carry it home (after paying for it, of course!). You may have been drawn in by the claims of rapid weight loss and fat-full delicious foods, but you may not be so sure about removing *all* carbohydrate foods — such as fruits and vegetables — entirely from your diet.

Well, look no further — this could well be the diet plan for you. Gone are the days of fruit-free diets and fatty steaks smothered in béarnaise sauce. Read on for a fully integrated diet plan that you can follow healthfully and deliciously for the rest of your life. Not only does it contribute to a healthy lifestyle, it will help you lose those extra pounds you may be carrying around.

About This Book

I originally designed a version of this low-carb eating plan for weight loss in our clinics at Texas Tech Medical Center. Unlike many other popular low-carb eating plans available today, this plan helps you control, *but doesn't entirely eliminate,* the intake of refined sugars and flour, and it encourages you to eat whole, unprocessed food. You may be surprised to see that the plan contains moderate amounts of starch, protein, and fat. That's because the plan allows your nutrition needs to be supplied *naturally.*

I help you focus your eating on natural, unprocessed foods whenever possible, particularly fresh fruits and vegetables, lean meat and protein, and low-fat dairy. I give you guidelines for appropriate serving sizes of carbohydrates. This is not the eat-all-the-fat-and-protein-you-can-stuff-in-your-face plan. But I have a whole chapter on free foods that you can eat anytime, anywhere, and in any quantity, so don't fret. You'll definitely feel full and energetic on this plan.

Conventions Used in This Book

Carbohydrates are counted differently in this plan than in other low-carb diets. Other low-carb diets count all the carbohydrate in a meal regardless of the food source. In this plan, you are given five carbohydrate choices per day. A carbohydrate choice is approximately 15 grams of total carbohydrate and can be a bread, cereal, starchy vegetable, pasta, chips, sugar, or sweet. In recipes, you only count the carbohydrate that comes from starch or sugar, not carbohydrate from fruit, vegetables, or low-fat dairy foods. Because of this difference, the recipes in this book have the number of carbohydrate choices calculated for you. That information will be stated in **bold.** The nutrition analysis of the recipes will calculate the total carbohydrate, but if that carbohydrate is supplied by fruit or vegetables and not starch or sugar, the recipe will be considered "free" and will be marked with a Green Light icon. For more information on this system, turn to Chapter 11.

The bottom line: When you see a Green Light icon next to a recipe, you know you can eat as much of it as you want. If the recipe doesn't have a Green Light icon, look to the Yield line to find out how many carbohydrate choices one serving of that recipe counts for, and plan your day accordingly.

Foolish Assumptions

This book is definitely a modified approach to low-carb dieting compared to many of the currently popular diet plans. But as such it is a much more successful plan over the long haul for most people. I am not completely eliminating sugar from your life. I am not asking you to count every floret of broccoli. I *am* looking at the overall quality of the carbohydrates that you put into your mouth and their effect on your body.

So here's a quick list of things that are different on this plan from what you might assume would be included in a low-carb dieting book:

- **You won't count every gram of carbohydrate you consume each day.** I do recommend a lower intake of carbohydrates, but I focus more on the *quality* of the carbohydrates. This is a departure from some on the low-carb side of the fence, but I believe it's the best choice for your long-term health. You'll eat as many green vegetables as you want, without counting carb grams. (Gasp!) But, you'll be limited on the amount of bread, cereal, and starchy vegetables you consume in a day. I show you how to gain control of the processed starches and sugar in your diet. For more on how this works, check out Part II — it's all there.

- **You will eat fruit.** So many low-carb diet plans remove fruit entirely from the plan. "An apple a day, keeps the doctor away" is not so far off. This plan encourages you to choose from an almost limitless list of fruits. In fact, I recommend fruit for its fiber, vitamins, and phytochemicals. You can eat fruit and still live a low-carb lifestyle, with all the benefits.

✔ **You will not eat as much fat as you want.** I focus on lean meats and low-fat dairy. I make a clear distinction between saturated fats and unsaturated fats and their effect on your health. As much as you may want unlimited amounts of hollandaise sauce to be good for you, it isn't. Fat is far from the culprit it was made out to be during the late '80s and early '90s, but that doesn't mean that unlimited quantities are good for you. Take a look at Chapter 8 for the real deal on fats.

✔ **You will not be hungry on this plan.** More accurately, there's no need to stay hungry on this plan. I don't want you to be hungry! You have pages upon pages of unlimited snacks to choose from, as well as recipe recommendations for spicing them up.

How This Book Is Organized

This book is divided into seven parts, all of which are described in the following sections.

Part I: Understanding the Carbohydrate Controversy

They say, "Those who ignore history are doomed to repeat it." In this part, I give you a peek at the substantial changes in the diet of the average American over the past 25 years that have contributed to increased obesity and chronic illnesses. I sort out both sides of the low-fat versus low-carb debate. I give you my approach to low-carb dieting for weight loss and a lifetime of good health. And most importantly, you can use this part to determine if low-carb eating is right for you.

Part II: Steering Yourself Back to Whole Foods

In this part, I detail the Whole Foods Eating Plan. I show you why all carbs aren't created equal and give you tips on the best carbohydrates to eat. I explain how to lower your overall carbohydrate intake *and* maintain a healthy lifestyle. You'll enjoy fruits, vegetables, and lean proteins — most whenever and in whatever quantities you want. You'll discover how to set reasonable limits on starchy carbs, good fats, and dairy products. I show you how you can navigate the Whole Foods Eating Plan for the rest of your life.

Part III: Shopping, Cooking, and Dining Out

In this part, I give you recipes and meal plans for guests or quick family suppers. I give you tips on make-ahead meals and treats so you're prepared for eating emergencies. I show you how to simplify your mornings without skipping breakfast, no matter how busy you are. I show you how to get in and out of the supermarket with low-carb-friendly foods without gouging your wallet. And I cover eating out (because we all do from time to time), the low-carb way.

Part IV: Recognizing Factors Other Than Food

Low-carb dieting can and should be a permanent lifestyle, and losing weight is only part of that equation. In this part I show you the whole range of health benefits, including reducing your risks of many obesity-related illnesses (like cardiovascular disease and diabetes), which you can achieve with gradual changes to your diet and lifestyle. Exercise is an important part of any health or weight-loss plan. In this part, I discuss the almost limitless benefits that daily exercise provides, including increased energy levels, better sleeping, and reduced stress. I also discuss vitamins and supplements and their appropriate role in low-carb dieting. Most of all, I help you set realistic, incremental goals for yourself, so you can look great and feel great, without beating yourself up.

Part V: Sticking to the Plan

Commitment is the cornerstone of any successful lifestyle change. One of the most intriguing aspects of low-carb dieting is that you get almost immediate gratification. Typically, energy levels increase quickly and weight comes off steadily, if you're committed. Despite this fact, as with any diet plan or lifestyle change, staying committed can be tough. Part V is loaded with tips and tricks to help you set yourself up to succeed with a low-carb lifestyle — as well as tips on how to forgive yourself when you fail. I help you analyze what went wrong in your plan and show you how to keep on keepin' on.

Part VI: The Part of Tens

You have questions; I have answers. Check out this part for a full list of commonly asked questions and a list of ways to track your progress (without a scale). And I've added quite a few additional resources in case you need additional or continuing support.

Part VII: Appendixes

In this part, I give you several excellent resources, like a grocery list — don't leave home without it. Other appendixes will come in handy at home when you're analyzing your progress. I put cross-references throughout the book whenever appropriate, so you know just what to do with each and every appendix.

Icons Used in This Book

Icons are those little pictures you'll find in the margins throughout this book. Here's a key to what they mean:

The Tip icon is very handy and used extensively in this book. It marks things that are sure to help you in your journey to lifelong good health. From cooking tips to exercise tips, it's all here and usually marked with this icon.

The Remember icon marks important points that are reinforced throughout a section of the book. You'll do well to remember what I point out here.

Because you've purchased this book, I know you care about your own health. Pay particular attention to the Warning icon to steer clear of situations that could be seriously dangerous or hazardous. Exercise some extra caution.

This little graphic marks information that is interesting but not essential for you to understand. You can even skip over the text here if it doesn't appeal to you and still enjoy the rest of the book. Sometimes it just marks the why's of a particular concept, so read and enjoy, but don't feel bogged down if you'd rather avoid it.

The Whole Foods icon marks info that's specific to the diet plan I've developed, rather than information about low-carb dieting in general. For a quick overview of the plan, take a look at Chapter 2, but watch for this icon throughout the book.

Green Light foods are free foods that you can eat anytime anywhere. They are primarily vegetables, fruits, lean meats, and low-fat cheeses. Green Light foods are covered extensively in Chapter 5 but are used throughout the book. Recipes using only these foods are marked with a Green Light icon so you'll know they're free.

Where to Go from Here

One of the best things about this book, or any *For Dummies* book for that matter, is the fact that you can start just about anywhere and find something that's interesting and relevant. So feel free to start wherever you want and move around at your leisure.

If you'd like a little more guidance, try this handy list on for size:

- ✔ If you'd like to get shopping right away and need a grocery list to get you started, go right to Appendix C.

- ✔ If you're not sure if the plan is right for you, take a look at Chapter 4. It's full of information on discovering your own personal health history, assessing your current health situation, and specifics on why this plan can work for you.

- ✔ If you want tips on eating out, the low-carb way, Chapter 13 is full of helpful information.

- ✔ To get straight to the recipes, focus on Chapters 11 and 12. Most are included there. For a quick list of which recipes I include in the book, take a look at the Recipes at a Glance at the front of the book.

- ✔ If you'd like a quick overview of the plan, and why it's better than any other low-carb plan out there, take a look at Chapter 2.

Part I

Understanding the Carbohydrate Controversy

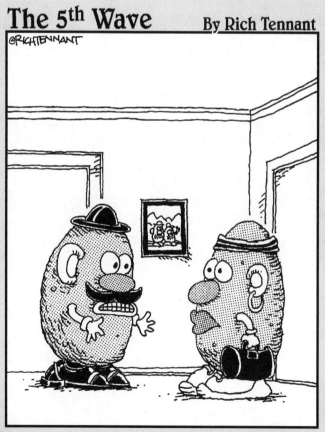

The 5th Wave   By Rich Tennant

"Look, you're never going to look like Mrs. French Fry, or Mrs. Cheese Stick. Besides, do you have any idea what their cholesterol levels are?"

In this part . . .

1 explain the controversy surrounding low-carbohydrate, high-protein diets and clarify the confusion. I sort out the good, the bad, and the ugly on both sides of the low-fat versus low-carb debate. I map out my approach to low-carb eating for a lifetime of good health. And most importantly, you'll have a chance to determine if lower-carb eating is right for you. You'll take a look at your own personal health story, the Body Mass Index, and assess your lifestyle to set realistic, attainable goals.

Chapter 1

Mapping Out Low-Carb Dieting

In This Chapter

▶ Understanding low-carb dieting

▶ Choosing the best carbs for your body

▶ Maintaining a low-carb lifestyle

*E*ating in America has changed. Americans eat out more frequently, eat larger portions of food, and eat more foods with little resemblance to their form in nature. As a result, more Americans than ever are overweight and struggling to find a weight-loss plan that lets them lose the extra pounds.

In this chapter, I map out a low-carb eating plan that is healthy *and* satisfying. I show you how to remove *refined carbohydrates* (carbohydrates with lots of sugar and very little fiber) from your diet, to make your diet healthier. By improving the quality of the carbohydrates you eat, and by controlling your daily intake of starchy carbs (like breads, pasta, and starchy vegetables), you'll lose weight and experience many other healthy benefits including increased energy, improved mood, and better sleeping.

To Eat Low-Carb or Low-Fat? That Is the Question

Currently, the debate rages between proponents of low-fat and low-carb diets. I'm sure you've heard the sound byte, "Fat makes you fat." Most Americans have gotten the low-fat dieting message. In fact, on average, Americans have reduced the percentage of fat in their diet to 33 percent of the calories they consume, as recommend by the low-fat experts. But even so, more than half of adult Americans are overweight. Our overall percentage of calories from fat went down, primarily because the actual number of calories we eat has gone up. We are eating more food than ever. Carbohydrate has replaced much of the fat in the American diet — and the increased food intake means an increased carbohydrate intake. This increased carbohydrate intake is largely sugars, sweeteners, and processed flour. The increase in carbohydrate from these refined sources has had a direct impact on the health (and waistlines) of Americans.

In working with overweight patients at Texas Tech Medical Center, I found a low-carb eating plan approach more effective than a low-fat diet approach. Patients watching their fat intake were eating a lot of fat-free food products that were not any healthier than the fat they had been eating.

What this diet is about

If you've looked into low-carb diets, you've probably found more than a few that require you to banish carbs from your diet entirely. And if you like carbs the way most people do, you've probably thrown down those books with a mixture of fear and frustration. Don't worry — the guidelines I give you in this book do *not* ask you to remove carbs from your diet completely. Instead, I want to get you thinking about the quality of the foods you consume, rather than the number of carb grams those foods contain. Rest assured that you will be allowed enough carb grams for good health, but I will do most of the counting for you. All you will need to do is choose delicious foods. For more details about this, turn to Chapter 2.

This is not an "eat-all-the-fat-and-protein-you-can-possibly-consume" diet. It's really focused on enjoying *whole* or *unprocessed foods* and enjoying the healthy side effects, including having more energy, stabilizing your blood-sugar levels, losing weight, and improving your self-confidence. (Whole foods are fruits, vegetables, grains, beans, nuts, and seeds that have not been processed to remove vitamins, minerals, fiber, and so on. They are foods that are sold to consumers in close to the same state that nature provided them.)

Most foods contain some carbohydrates. Even an 8-ounce glass of skim milk contains 12 grams of carbs. A cup of broccoli contains 8 carb grams. And yet, both milk and broccoli are packed full of other nutritional benefits, including vitamins, nutrients, fiber, and phytochemicals. If you strictly limit the number of carb grams in your diet without considering the *quality* of the carbs you eat, you'll be missing out on some key foods that will enhance your overall good health.

On this low-carb plan, you'll be limited to five carbohydrate servings a day, but many foods that contain carbohydrates are absolutely *free* (which on this diet means you can have as many of them as you want, without counting them toward your daily carb allowance). Check out Chapters 5 and 6 for the full scoop on which carbs fall into which categories, but here are some quick tips on which foods to focus your attention on and which to pass by:

> ✔ **Don't be afraid of fruit.** Fruit does contain carbohydrates, but the carbs in fruit give it a delicious *natural* sweetness, which is partnered with a ton of vitamins, fiber, and relatively few calories. Increasing your fruit intake is a great way to help you wean yourself off *refined sugars* (refined

sugars are sugars like table sugar and high-fructose corn syrup that are added to processed foods). Fruits make a great dessert option and, because they come pre-portioned in their own natural package, they're a great choice for grab-and-go snacks. On this diet plan, almost all fruits are *free* (meaning you can eat as many of them as you like). For more on free foods (and which fruits *aren't* free), see Chapter 5.

✔ **Look at leafy green and non-starchy vegetables.** Leafy greens, like spinach, watercress, cabbage, and romaine lettuce, and non-starchy vegetables, like green beans, broccoli, carrots, and tomatoes, come in an almost limitless variety. You can further vary your diet by trying new preparations of old favorites and partnering them with new choices. Check out some great recipes for salads and other greens in Chapter 5.

✔ **Remove refined sugars from your life.** Refined sugars provide calories, but lack vitamins, minerals, and fiber. The amount of refined sugar in the American diet is a disastrous, but fairly recent, development. Watch out for hidden sugars in breads, lunch meat, and salad dressings. Pay attention to the not-hidden sugars in non-diet sodas, cookies, and candy. For more on reducing the amount of sugar in your diet, see Chapter 6.

And, for those five carbohydrate servings you're allowed to eat each day, choose the following:

✔ **Check out legumes.** *Legumes* (leh-GOOMS) are foods like peas, beans, and peanuts. They are nutritional powerhouses that add fiber to your diet, are naturally low in fat, are a great source of protein, and are very inexpensive. Look for several varieties at your market including canned, dried, and fresh. Legumes make great additions to salads, serve as excellent side dishes, and make healthy delicious entrees in their own right. Look for great recipes for legumes throughout Parts II and III of this book.

✔ **Choose whole grains whenever possible.** Look for *whole grains* (grains that still have their bran and nutrients intact) as the first ingredient on a food nutrition label's ingredients list. Items made from whole grains tend to be higher in fiber, lower in sugar, and have a stabilizing affect on blood sugar levels compared to their refined-grain counterparts. For more on the benefits of fiber and whole grains, take a look at Chapter 6.

✔ **Introduce more soy products into your diet.** Soy foods contain both carbs and protein, making them off-limits on many low-carb eating plans. Not so with my plan. In fact, if you're a vegetarian, you can substitute soy products for lean proteins in your diet and still get many of the nutritional benefits this plan has to offer. Regardless of whether you're a vegetarian, adding more soy to your diet can offer tremendous health benefits, including a reduced risk of several types of cancer and heart disease, as well as more-balanced hormone levels. Check out Chapter 6 for more good news about soy products.

Whether low-carb eating is right for you

Take a good look at Chapter 4 to determine if low-carb dieting is right for you. But for now, the following are *all* good reasons to follow this low-carb plan:

- ✔ If your personal health history includes the precursors to diabetes, high blood pressure, or heart disease
- ✔ If you're concerned about stabilizing your blood sugar levels
- ✔ If you're tired of the way convenience foods and prepackaged, sugar-laden foods make you feel
- ✔ If your Body Mass Index (BMI) is 30 or above (turn to Appendix A to determine your BMI)

Be sure to check with your personal healthcare practitioner before beginning any exercise or diet regimen.

Discovering Whole Foods

The most important element of the eating plan I cover in this book is the introduction of whole foods into your diet. A *whole food* is any food that's not refined or processed. Fresh, frozen, or canned fruits and vegetables are whole foods; French fries are not. A sirloin steak is a whole food; a breaded veal cutlet is not. Whole-grain bread is a whole food; white bread is not. Apple juice is a whole food; a fruit roll-up is not. A baked potato is a whole food; potato chips are not.

The more refined a food is, the fewer vitamins and nutrients and the less fiber the food has. If you see a food that's refined but has been fortified with vitamins and minerals, like sugary breakfast cereal, be wary. These vitamins aren't as easily used by your body for all of its vital processes as their naturally occurring counterparts. And 99 times out of 100, the food contains more sugar than your body needs.

Check out Part II for the skinny on using whole foods to their best dietary advantage.

Living the Low-Carb Way

Low-carb dieting will become second nature to you quickly. The key to your success is planning. Plan your meals and plan your shopping trips to fit with your low-carb lifestyle. You can minimize impulse buys by having a plan to stick to.

Be aware of the layout of your grocery store. Food manufacturers want to lure you toward the center aisles of the grocery store where the shelves are stocked with expensive prepared dinners and other refined foods. Stick to the perimeter of the grocery store for most whole-food choices (such as fresh produce, low-fat dairy products, and lean meats). When you do take the plunge into the center aisles for dried beans, canned vegetables, or whole oats, avoid the temptation to toss prepackaged dinner helpers, chips, cookies, or sugary cereals into your cart. For more shopping tips, take a look at Chapter 9.

With a little effort, you'll be able to navigate your way around a low-carb kitchen. My pantry tends to be full of canned whole veggies rather than canned soup, which typically contains more sodium and modified food starch than vegetables. I use fresh or frozen beef, canned beans, and tomatoes to make my own chili instead of buying premade canned chili. Find your own shortcuts to make your life easier *and* low-carb friendly.

When dining out, don't be afraid to ask for substitutions. If your steak comes with French fries, ask for an extra side of veggies instead. If the pasta special sounds very tempting, the chef can likely make it for you without the pasta. Just think of that chunky seafood in a hearty marinara sauce — it's fantastic without the white pasta. Most restaurants, even fast-food restaurants, have a house or green salad that's a great addition to any meal and totally free on this eating plan. Just get your dressing on the side, so you don't eat unwanted fat and calories. For more tips on dining out, skip ahead to Chapter 13.

Beyond the Scale: Identifying Other Factors for Overall Health

For most people, weight loss and dieting go hand in hand. In fact, when you hear someone say, "I'm on a diet," it usually means, "I'm trying to lose weight." But the word *diet* (coming from the Latin *dieta,* or "daily regimen") can also refer simply to the food you eat day in and day out. I want to change your daily food plan for the rest of your life, not just help you lose weight now. So, considering factors other than a number on the scale is important when you're charting your progress.

Lowering your Body Mass Index (BMI), or body fat percentage, by as few as two points can have a profoundly positive effect on your overall health. Check out Chapter 3 and Appendix A for details.

Your body shape, genetics, and age have as much to do with your physical appearance as your weight. So set realistic expectations for what you expect your body to look like. An unrealistic self-image can be devastating to your health and self-esteem. For more details, take a look at Chapter 15.

Exercise and low-carb dieting: Your partners in fitness

Exercise isn't just a necessary part of life, it's fun! With so many different forms of exercise available, you're sure to find one that matches your interests and lifestyle. You don't have to run out and buy Spandex, join a gym, and attend a Pilates class this week. Just pulling weeds in the garden or mowing the lawn can get your heart pumping. Walk around the block with your dog. Find a friend to walk with you during your lunch break. Volunteer to coach a Little League team in the sport of your choice. Anything that gets you moving is a great addition to your lifestyle.

The effects of exercise are cumulative, which means that you don't have to get your 30 minutes a day in one shot. You can take a 15-minute walk around the block in the morning, and another 15-minute walk after dinner.

Daily exercise stabilizes your blood sugar levels, improves your cardiovascular health, increases your strength and stamina, and helps you get a better night of sleep. You may feel more tired immediately after beginning a new exercise program, but you should quickly enjoy increased energy levels, as well as an improved mood because of the *endorphins* running rampant in your bloodstream.

Endorphins are chemical signals in your blood that act like your body's own version of morphine or painkillers. Production of endorphins in the body is linked to increased exercise and produces a feeling of euphoria, sometimes labeled as *runner's high* in athletes. After exercise, the endorphins improve your sense of well-being.

The more you exercise, the more lean muscle you develop. And the more lean muscle you develop, the higher your resting *metabolism.* (Your metabolism is sort of your internal rhythm, or the rate at which you burn calories when completely at rest.) With a higher resting metabolism, you burn more calories while you're sleeping, working at your desk, or even just breathing. How's that for efficiency?

Exploring vitamins and supplements

On the Whole Foods Eating Plan, you're encouraged to take in most of your vitamins and minerals through the whole foods that you consume. However, a few important exceptions may exist. If you're at risk for osteoporosis, you'll want to calculate your calcium intake, and if it doesn't meet your daily need, add a calcium supplement to your daily regimen. Certain health conditions and certain stages in life may make considering a vitamin or mineral supplement appropriate as well. Antioxidant nutrients like vitamins C, E, and beta-carotene and the minerals zinc, copper, selenium, and manganese may help lower your risk of disease and the ravages of aging. New guidelines for supplements and information on upper limits can help you to know the amounts to take and still stay within safe levels.

For more on incorporating vitamins and supplements into your low-carb lifestyle, take a look at Chapter 14 and Appendix D.

Maintaining Your Low-Carb Lifestyle

As with making any long-term change to your diet, the key to enjoying the ultimate benefits of your low-carb lifestyle is sticking with the plan. Part V is loaded with tips and tricks to help you set yourself up to succeed.

Making the commitment

The first step in making the low-carb commitment is mental or psychological. Customize your food habits to meet the demands of your lifestyle and your low-carb diet. If you can get your family, roommates, or other housemates to follow the diet with you, you'll definitely have a better shot at success, because you can completely remove tempting foods and sweets from your cabinets and fridge. But don't stress if others aren't interested in the plan. You can still cook for the whole family with the plan and adjust your own portion sizes to coincide with it. You'll just need to be careful not to indulge in cookies or snacks. For more on getting (and staying) committed to the plan, check out Chapters 16 and 17.

Planning ahead

Let your lifestyle help determine your food-plan strategy. If you know that you have no time in the mornings, prepare your healthy breakfast and lunch the night before. Plan your meals before you're hungry. Making healthy choices is much more difficult when you're hungry and refined foods are handy.

The rise of prepackaged, convenience foods has increased the amount of refined sugar in the American diet, but your busy schedule doesn't have to be a barrier to healthy eating. Keep healthy snacks on hand in snack-size resealable plastic bags for easy treats. You'll eliminate the urge to grab cookies, chips, and crackers.

Cook meals in quantity. Roast a large turkey or ham for lots of leftovers and soups or salads. Double entree sizes so you can eat one and freeze one for later. Buy reusable plastic containers that go from freezer to microwave for your own frozen lunch entrees. For more planning tips, check out Chapters 10 and 17.

Picking yourself up when you fall

I wish I could say that no one ever slips up on this plan, that no one ever gives in to temptation and succumbs to that extra baked potato or slice of cake. But the fact is giving in to temptation is part of life. You're human and, therefore, you aren't perfect. However, don't beat up on yourself when you slip up, and more importantly, don't use it as an excuse to throw all your progress out the window. So you had a piece of cake and didn't save any carb choices for it? Analyze what went wrong in your plan and resolve to have a better day tomorrow. These small setbacks can be the gateway to long-term success. If you can learn from them and make better choices in the same situation next time, you can have better overall health and weight control. For specifics on getting it together (again), take a look at Chapter 18.

Chapter 2

The Great Debate: Carbs versus Fat

*N*othing has polarized the nutrition world as much as the low-carbohydrate diet, but the low-carb diet isn't new. It's been around for over 100 years — and for most of that time, it has been controversial. The quick-weight-loss effect of the low-carb diet, its permission to eat as much meat and fat as you want, and the lack of hunger in those who follow it has always attracted many fans. However, very-low-carb diets have a short lifespan.

In this chapter, I show you why the low-carb diet is controversial. I discuss the migration of the American diet toward more calories from increased snacks, sugars, soft drinks, and bigger portions of all foods. I give you ways to evaluate low-carb diet plans to help you make the best choice for you. And most importantly, I give you an overview of the Whole Foods Eating Plan, which is healthy for a lifetime and will also help you lose excess pounds.

Evaluating the Controversy

The low-carb diet gained modern-day popularity about 30 years ago only to later be squelched by the fully accepted and heavily promoted low-fat diet. Cholesterol was implicated as a major determinant of heart disease, and diets high in saturated fat were found to raise blood cholesterol levels. Lowering fat intake in the diet enjoyed approval by the scientific community and was embraced by national health organizations and public policy. There was a halo-effect over the low-fat diet and horns and a devil's fork over fat. Fat was branded as the ultimate dietary villain, for several reasons:

- ✔ Heart disease was increasing and was correlated with high cholesterol. Scientists discovered that saturated fat increased cholesterol levels in the blood. It was also sensed that people were slowly becoming a little fatter. A fat gram contained twice the number of calories of protein or carbohydrate grams, so a good way to reduce the number of calories we ate was to reduce the number of fat grams we consumed.

- ✔ Fat was also blamed for cancer and a host of other diseases.

The low-fat diet pranced around the arena as having delivered the ultimate knock-out to the low-carbohydrate diet.

Then, about eight years ago, the low-carbohydrate diet started coming up from the mat and came on with a vengeance. Media headlines questioned the honesty of the low-fat diet, and nutrition scientists were accused of waffling on their nutrition advice. The low-fat diet was knocked on its heels and struggled to stay in the ring. Obesity was worse than ever, now at epidemic proportions; cancer was also just as bad as ever. Both were accompanied by increases in diabetes, high blood pressure, joint pain, and heartburn. Heartburn became more sophisticated and was renamed gastroesophageal reflux disease (GERD) and a "new" disease phenomena had appeared on the scene dastardly labeled as *Syndrome X* or *metabolic syndrome.* Metabolic syndrome is considered a strong risk factor for heart disease. (Check out Chapter 4 for more information on metabolic syndrome.) Accusing fingers pointed directly at carbohydrate as the villain. The low-fat diet, which recommended carbohydrate as a substitute for fat, was dealt a blow. Even the United States Department of Agriculture's Food Pyramid was included as an enabler. The low-carb diet started a victory dance.

So, where is the truth? Is it the very-low-fat diet? No. Is it the very-low-carb diet? No. Do we need to eat less fat? Yes. Do we need to eat less carbohydrate? Yes. In fact, we need to eat less of just about everything.

The low-fat, high-carb diet

Americans are heavier than ever before, despite the fact that they're reducing the percentage of calories consumed from fat. Popular diet books and the media immediately targeted carbohydrates as the bad guys and labeled them fattening. What was ignored is the fact that in 1994 the average American consumed 40,000 calories more (over the course of a year) than they did in 1990. The real message should be that excess calories from *any* source will result in increased body weight. High-carbohydrate diets recommend that the carbohydrate comes from fruits, vegetables, beans, whole grains, and dairy, but high-carb diets also impose a tight restriction on fat.

The history of the low-carb diet

The low-carb diet is not new. In fact, it was devised by a London coffin maker and undertaker named William Banting to treat his own obesity. He had become so obese that he had to walk downstairs backwards to keep from falling. He lost 50 pounds on the diet and published a pamphlet, *Letter on Corpulence, Addressed to the Public,* in 1864. Banting declared the diet a "cure for extreme corpulence." His cure became so popular that the word *banting* became a synonym for dieting in the English language. The diet also caught the interest of Americans in the late 1800s and became popular. However, in the next century, it was labeled the "Banting Scheme" because it was full of unproven medical lingo and followers of the plan often developed gout. Since those early days, the low-carb diet approach has resurfaced about every 25 years and is always controversial.

One thing the advocates of the low-fat diet didn't plan on was the abundance of fat-free foods that would become available. The low-fat message became distorted into counting fat grams. Therefore, *fat-free* foods just became *free* foods in people's minds. The fat in sweet rolls, cookies, cake, and crackers was replaced with sugar or other refined sweeteners. USDA food consumption data verifies that the intake of sugar and sweeteners increased 25 percent between 1970 and 1995. Intake of fruits, vegetables, beans, and grains, the preferred replacement for fat, increased some, but it still fell short of the recommended goals.

The low-carb, high-protein diet

With carbohydrate at an all-time high and the health of the country as bad as ever, the low-carbohydrate diet rose in favor. People following the low-carb diet attest to its effectiveness and proudly proclaim the number of pounds lost. So if it's effective in losing weight as so many contend, then what's the problem?

Most low-carb diets count grams of carbohydrate regardless of the food source. So "good" carbs, such as fruit, vegetables, whole grains, and dairy, are eliminated solely because they contain carbohydrate. If you follow these restrictions, you're eliminating vital nutrients, phytochemicals, and fiber (see Chapter 3). Certainly, everyone needs to eat less carbohydrate, but the decrease needs to come mainly from refined flour and sugar products. You must take into consideration the *quality* of the carbohydrate you eat.

Another problem is that low-carb diets tend to be high in fat and protein. Many interpret the low-carb diet as a license to load up on bun-less burgers, steaks, sausages, eggs, and bacon. Unfortunately, this approach can have potentially negative health effects.

Whether you count grams of fat or count grams of carbohydrate, you're still using a calculator to make your food choices. Give me a break! Who wants to eat a calculator? Counting all fats the same and counting all carbohydrates the same is misleading. You should definitely include some fats in your diet and you should definitely include some carbohydrates. For the full story on fats, take a peek at Chapter 8. For the lowdown on quality carbs, see Chapters 5 and 6.

Where We Went Wrong: Deconstructing the Typical (Bad) Diet

The modern diet includes more calories, larger portion sizes, and increased frequency of eating. The modern American diet is characterized by all the following:

- More soft drinks and sweeteners
- More salty snacks
- More cookies and snack foods
- Eating out more often, especially in fast-food restaurants
- Larger portion sizes, especially of soft drinks and French fries
- Increased convenience, microwaveable, and processed foods

Instead of the USDA Food Guide Pyramid, the modern diet looks like what you see in Figure 2-1.

Eating more refined sugars

Most of the increase in sugar in the American diet has come from *added sugars*. Added sugars are sugars and syrups added to foods in processing or preparation, not the naturally occurring sugars in foods like fructose in fruit or lactose in milk. Sugar (including sucrose, corn sweeteners, honey, maple syrup, and molasses) is everywhere in the foods we eat — and it's often hidden. Sugar is the number-one food additive and turns up in some unlikely places like pizza, bread, hot dogs, boxed mixed rice, soup, crackers, spaghetti sauce, lunchmeat, canned vegetables, fruit drinks, flavored yogurt, ketchup, salad dressings, mayonnaise, and some peanut butter.

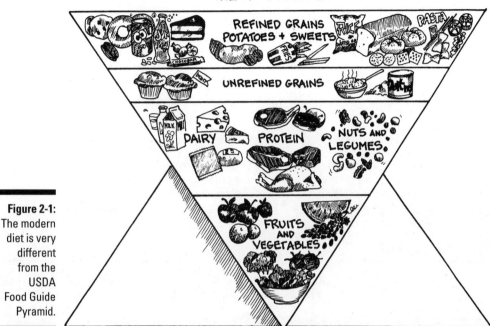

THE MODERN DIET

The number-one food source containing added sugar consumed in the United States is soft drinks, including non-diet soda or pop. Carbonated sodas provided about 30 percent of the refined and added sugars in the American food supply, compared with 16 percent in 1970. Over 50 percent of American adults, 65 percent of teenage girls, and 74 percent of teenage boys consume soft drinks daily, most of which are sugar-sweetened rather than artificially sweetened. Intake of a lot of foods high in added sugars, especially soft drinks, is of concern especially in children, teenagers, and women because, when people are drinking soft drinks, they're not drinking as much of the nutritious foods like milk.

Other significant sources of added sugar in the American diet include candy, cakes, cookies, pies, fruitades and drinks (such as fruit punch and lemonade), and dairy desserts (such as ice cream).

Eating more salty snacks

According to information from a national food consumption survey, the intake of salty snack foods in 1978 was 17.5 pounds per person per year. In 1994 the intake was 22 pounds per person per year. This is an increase of about 5 pounds of snack foods per person! This means that everyone is eating the equivalent of a small bag of chips every day. If I don't eat *any,* that means someone else is eating *two* small bags of chips every day. Twenty years ago, snack foods were about 11 percent of the diet, but by 1996 that had increased to 17 percent. Another study indicates that salty snack food intake has doubled in the past 20 years. In addition to extra salt, snack foods provide calories from refined grains and sugar. They contribute little nutritional value and displace more nutritious fruits and vegetables in the diet.

Eating more fast foods

Eating in fast-food restaurants is so pervasive that, to increase profits, fast-food companies have to work to get customers away from other fast-food restaurants rather than bring in customers who are completely new to fast food. What does this mean? Virtually *everyone* eats at fast-food restaurants at least occasionally.

The fructose story

Americans and their children have become high consumers of sugar and sweet-tasting foods and beverages. Caloric sweeteners, most notably high-fructose corn syrup, have dramatically increased in the past 20 or so years. High-fructose corn syrup is predominantly used in soft drinks (check the label the next time you drink one), but it's also found in frozen foods, bakery foods, and vending machine products.

Before 1970, high-fructose corn syrup was unknown in the food supply. It was developed in the 1970s as an economical way to produce a cheaper sweetener for commercial use. It is six times sweeter than cane sugar and is produced from corn, which gives food manufacturers a way to sweeten food products at a significant cost savings. By the end of the 1970s, mass-production techniques had been developed to make its use widespread.

Currently, high-fructose corn syrup makes up over 40 percent of our excessively high sugar intake. Fructose was once thought to be used by the body just like sucrose (table sugar). It's now known that high concentrations of fructose are metabolized differently. Due to this difference, ingesting high concentrations of fructose can increase the likelihood of weight gain and its associated insulin resistance. In addition to obesity, insulin resistance results in glucose intolerance, high triglyceride levels, high blood pressure, and increased risk of diabetes and heart disease.

The current levels of soft drink and sweetened food intake is an aspect of the modern lifestyle unknown in the past. The inclusion of high-fructose corn syrup in the food supply parallels the dramatic increase in obesity, diabetes, and insulin resistance. Sweet-tasting foods in the diet stimulate a craving for more sweet foods, which can lead to overconsumption. Low-carbohydrate diets have the advantage of reducing the intake of soft drinks and foods with high-fructose corn sweeteners, but they don't deal with the desire many Americans have for sweet tastes.

In 1996, Americans ate 8 million more orders of French fries, almost 6 million more hamburgers, and 5 million more servings of fried-chicken nuggets than they did in 1995 — and that was seven years ago (which means we're most likely eating even more today). A low-fat hamburger was dropped from a popular fast-food chain due to poor sales — so apparently Americans aren't buying the low-fat approach when they're eating fast food.

Eating larger portion sizes

A recent study compared the portions of popular foods to USDA and Food and Drug Administration (FDA) standards. The typical cookie is *700 percent larger* than the USDA suggested size. Most people eat a single serving of pasta that is 480 percent larger than recommended. And the average muffin exceeds the standard by 333 percent.

Portion sizes in restaurants started to increase in the 1970s, grew dramatically in the 1980s, and currently continue to rise in parallel to increases in average American body weight. Restaurants long ago switched to a 12-inch dinner plate from the standard 10-inch plate. Studies show that Americans ignore portion sizes even when attempting to follow a healthy diet and will eat as much food as they're given. As a rule, they won't leave food on their plates.

When a popular fast-food chain opened in 1950, it sold only one size of regular French fries, containing 200 calories. In 1970, the regular French fries were then called "small" and a new "large" French fries containing 320 calories appeared on the menu. In 1980, the 320-calorie French fries were called "regular" and a newer "large" French fries containing 400 calories appeared on the menu. In 1990, the "large" French fries had grown to 450 calories and a new "super-size" French fries containing 540 calories appeared on the menu. And in 2000, the 540-calorie fry became "large" and a newer "super-size" French fries containing 610 calories appeared on the menu. Small and regular French fries are nowhere to be found on the menu. You can choose from medium, large, or super-sized. The kid meals come with the 320-calorie-sized fries.

Value meals and "super-sized" meals are a financial incentive for many eating establishments. They can add large-sized drinks and fries to a meal at minimal cost to them but increased cost to the consumer. So, in terms of nutritional quality, who gets the value from the "value" meal? Not you.

Eating more calories

Americans are starting the 21st century consuming more food and several hundred more calories per person per day than did their counterparts in the late 1950s when calorie consumption was at the lowest level in the last century. USDA-adjusted calorie intake data for the year 2000 indicated that the approximate calorie intake per person per day was 2,700. This is about

530 calories *more* per day than in 1970. About 47 percent of this increase comes from refined carbohydrates like processed grains and sugars, 37 percent from fats, and the remaining 16 percent from fruits, vegetables, meats, nuts, dairy products, and eggs.

Getting a lower percentage of calories from fat

The USDA food consumption survey revealed that the *percent of calories from fat* in the American diet continues to go down: 40 percent in the 1970s, 34 percent in 1990, and 33 percent in 1994. However, the *total number of calories consumed,* primarily from refined-carbohydrate foods, has increased. When the calories increase and the fat intake stays the same, the percent of calories from fat goes down. But the total amount in terms of actual grams of fat consumed per day has stayed about the same: Americans consumed 73 grams of fat per day in 1994 versus 72 grams of fat in 1990.

Even though the amount of fat consumed is about the same, more of the fat intake is represented by *trans fats.* Many processed carbohydrate foods contain trans fats from partially hydrogenated vegetable oils. Trans fats act like saturated fat by boosting levels of bad cholesterol and increasing the risk of heart disease. Trans fats are commonly found in carbohydrate foods such as cookies, crackers, chips, French fries, and fast foods.

Eating fewer fruits and vegetables

Fruit and vegetable consumption has increased, but still falls below recommended levels. In 1994, less than 10 percent of the American population ate the recommended five fruits and vegetables each day. The popularity of pizza in the 1990s boosted the average consumption of canned tomato products, but consumption of other canned vegetables declined. The popularity of French fries, eaten mainly in fast-food restaurants, caused a 63 percent increase in the average consumption of frozen potatoes. And the introduction of precut and prepackaged items has boosted the intake of fresh fruits and vegetables.

Highly publicized medical research linking compounds in fruits and vegetables to anticancer activity has provided a powerful incentive to consumption. However, in 1995 one fast-food company spent $800 million to promote its products, while the National Cancer Institute was only able to spend $1 million to promote fruits and vegetables. And consider the fact that that was only *one* fast-food company!

Go to Chapter 3 to find out more about the great diversity in carbohydrate foods.

Eating fewer whole grains

Individual use of flour and cereal products reached 200 pounds per person in 2000, up from 138 pounds in 1970. Unfortunately, most of this was in the form of refined flour food products and not in whole-grain food products. Refined flour products can quickly spike your blood sugar and overstimulate your insulin production. Whole-grain food products raise blood-sugar levels gradually without overstimulating insulin. This effect is important in controlling obesity, diabetes, and heart disease. New nutrition guidelines carry a strong recommendation to include at least three servings of whole-grain food products per day. According to a 1996 USDA survey, only 7 percent of Americans ate the recommended three or more servings of whole-grain foods a day.

Looking at the Nation's Health

With the changes that have occurred in the American food intake, the deterioration in the nation's health should come as no surprise. But food intake is not the only thing to blame; lack of exercise is a major contributor as well (see Chapter 15 for more on exercise). The American lifestyle is killing us — check out the following sections for information on how.

Obesity

Obesity has been growing rapidly in the past 20 years, but health officials were shocked by a 1999 study that revealed that 61 percent of the population is either overweight or obese. Obesity is linked to diabetes, heart disease, hypertension, osteoarthritis, and cancer. The effects of obesity cost Americans $100 billion per year.

Diabetes

Obesity is a worldwide epidemic and is being followed by a worldwide epidemic of diabetes. Seventeen million Americans have diabetes and 16 million more are at increased risk of developing the disease. People who are obese have a five times greater risk of developing diabetes than people who are of a normal weight.

Diabetes is a major health problem in the United States. It is characterized by an inability to keep blood-sugar levels consistent. There are two types of diabetes: Type 1, formerly called *juvenile diabetes,* requires insulin to keep blood-sugar levels consistent; type 2 diabetes, formerly called *maturity-onset* or *adult-onset diabetes,* does not require insulin. Type 2 diabetes is preceded by obesity and a condition called *insulin resistance.* Over 60 percent of the money spent on type 2 diabetes is due to obesity.

Syndrome X: Metabolic Syndrome

Syndrome X is a name coined for a modern disease characterized by obesity, glucose intolerance, high triglycerides, and high blood pressure. It has also been called Metabolic Syndrome, the Deadly Quartet, Insulin Resistance Syndrome, and pre-diabetes. *Insulin resistance* is the condition that causes this cluster of symptoms. Insulin resistance is a condition in which the body does not respond very well to the insulin it produces. (Insulin is a hormone that moves glucose out of the blood and into the tissues where it can be used.) If a person is insulin resistant, then he has to produce a greater amount of insulin in order to move the glucose into the tissue. High levels of insulin not only promote storage of fat but can cause serious harm to body organs. High levels of insulin cause high blood pressure, abnormal choles-terol levels, *atherosclerosis* (hardening of the arteries), and blood-clotting dis-orders. This can result in heart attacks and strokes. Eating high-carb foods — especially refined starchy and sugary foods — produces higher-than-normal amounts of insulin. The low-fat, high-carb diet universally recommended for high cholesterol is the worst diet for people who are insulin resistant. Check out Chapter 4 for more information on Syndrome X.

Turn to Chapter 4 for help in determining whether you are at risk for develop-ing insulin resistance.

Polycystic ovarian syndrome

Polycystic ovarian syndrome (PCOS) is an insulin-resistant disease in women that has become more prevalent in the past 20 years. PCOS is characterized by elevated levels of male hormone, increased facial hair, irregular menstrual periods, and infertility. It is the most common cause of female hormone dys-function and infertility. Women with PCOS may benefit from a low-carb diet.

Heart disease

The importance of insulin resistance as a heart disease risk factor has been rec-ognized. New treatment guidelines for the prevention of heart disease identify the cluster of abnormalities associated with insulin resistance as risk factors. Specifically, levels of *triglycerides* (a fat in the blood) have been added to the list of risk factors. High levels of triglycerides in your blood are not only related to your fat intake, but also to your intake of excess calories and carbohydrate.

High blood pressure

High blood pressure is one of the nation's leading health problems. Twenty-five percent of adults are known to have high blood pressure and an estimated 50 million are at risk of developing it. High blood pressure greatly raises the risk of stroke, heart failure, and kidney disease. New guidelines are urging Americans to make diet and exercise changes designed to lower their blood pressure. Seventy percent of high blood pressure is caused by obesity.

Compared with individuals with normal blood pressure, people with high blood pressure are relatively glucose intolerant. Insulin resistance is also a contributing factor to high blood pressure.

Arthritis and related conditions

Arthritis is a very common degenerative joint disease. It commonly affects the weight-bearing joints in the knees, hips, and lower back. The most common risk factors are obesity and a family history of the condition. Being obese causes increase wear and tear on the joints which decreases your ability to walk or get up and down out of a chair. There are different forms of arthritis and excess weight affects them all. Arthritis and joint conditions related to obesity are estimated to cost over $4 billion a year in health care.

Cancer

Consumption of excess calories, regardless of the source, increases the risk of breast, prostate, and colon cancer. But just as important is what we *don't* eat. Diets full of whole foods such as fruits, vegetables, beans, whole grains, and low-fat dairy products are known to lower cancer risk. Dietary patterns that provide only the minimum servings of these foods increase cancer risk.

Gastroesophageal reflux disease

Sometimes referred to as heartburn, gastroesophageal reflux disease (GERD) is much more extensive than heartburn. It has increased in incidence primarily due to obesity and the overconsumption of food. The intake of carbonated beverages and fatty and spicy foods aggravate the condition.

Is Low-Carb Dieting Dangerous?

The question of safety has always arisen in regard to low-carb diets. This is because some low-carb diet plans restrict *all* carbohydrate foods from the diet. Eliminating carbohydrate from your diet is almost impossible, but some diets require you to get down to 10 or 20 grams of carbs per day. In these kinds of severe carbohydrate restrictions, there is not only a restriction of vital nutrients from the diet there is also a loss of vital nutrients from the body. And as you can guess, when you lose vital nutrients, you can end up in poor health. Modern-day proponents of very-low-carb diets recognize this problem and are adamant in recommending vitamin and mineral supplements to cover the losses. Now think about it: Can a diet plan that requires supplements to replace lost nutrients from food be good? My plan doesn't completely eliminate carbs from your diet. In fact, you must eat some carbohydrates, like those found in fresh fruits and vegetables, to maintain good health. There's no way to get the necessary fiber, vitamins, and minerals, on a regular basis without some carbs. I'll show you how to pick the best and leave the rest.

Evaluating limits on carbs

A very-low-carb diet is any diet that requires less than 50 grams of carbohydrate per day. Eating a healthy diet on this level of carbohydrate restriction is impossible. If you tried, you'd be eliminating too many foods rich in vitamins, minerals, fiber, and cancer-fighters. Getting essential nutrients from foods is always better than getting it from supplements.

A moderately low-carbohydrate diet — such as this one — includes 100 to 150 grams of carbohydrate per day. Recent nutrition guidelines say that 130 grams of carbohydrate per day is the minimum level needed for adequate brain function in children and adults. This is also the minimum level to prevent loss of lean tissue from muscles and organs.

If you count the carbohydrate in milk, fruits, vegetables, legumes, breads, and cereals, 130 grams of carbohydrate would be provided by two servings of milk, two servings of fruit, three servings of vegetables, and four servings of legumes, breads, or cereals.

A high-carb diet, on the other hand, includes more than 250 grams of carbohydrate each day. This is appropriate for active people who are at a healthy weight (with a BMI between 20 and 25 — see Appendix A for more on BMI). No matter how many grams of carbs you eat every day, fruits, vegetables, whole grains, legumes, and pasta should be the main food sources of carbohydrates, with added sugar sources kept to a minimum.

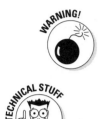

The potential physical consequences of very-low-carbohydrate diets range from mild to serious to life-threatening. Because the approach I recommend is a modified low-carbohydrate diet, you shouldn't experience any of these problems. But, as with any diet plan, consult your healthcare practitioner for advice before beginning the plan. Check out Chapter 3 for the physical consequences of very-low-carbohydrate diets.

Knowing how low-carb diets work

Removing carbohydrates from the diet drastically lowers your total caloric intake. (You may not realize that when you're chomping on that bunless cheeseburger or potato-less steak.) The low carbohydrate intake (or just lower calories) requires your body to break down glycogen from the liver and muscles to free glucose. *Glycogen* is glucose stored in your muscles and liver. Amino acids from the protein in your diet and in your muscles can be converted to glucose, but this is more difficult for your body than breaking down glycogen. Glycogen contains a lot of water and converting it to glucose releases the water. What does that mean for you? You'll urinate more frequently to get rid of the water.

After 7 to 14 days, the water loss ends and the phase of rapid weight loss slows down. If the carbohydrate intake is below 50 grams per day, then fat will be burned as fuel-producing ketones in your blood. (Ketones are the chemical byproduct of your body burning off fat for fuel.) Your body will get rid of the ketones through your kidneys. Usually very-low-carbohydrate diets encourage eight glasses of water a day. This is to help flush the ketones out of the body through the kidneys and to prevent dehydration. The high level of ketones in your blood also suppresses your appetite so you aren't as hungry. This helps people stay on the diet longer. The more overweight a person is when she starts the diet, the greater the initial weight loss. Of course, this is also very encouraging, but

remember that the weight loss is more water loss than fat loss.

Carbohydrate foods represent a great portion of a person's food intake. They are foods most people like to eat. Eventually, when people have been restricting their carbohydrate intake severely, they reintroduce carbs to their diet. Actually, some people do that by "cheating" on the diet. I routinely hear people say that the reason they like the low-carbohydrate diet is because they can cheat on it and still lose weight. Now, that cheating those people are talking about doesn't occur with fruits and vegetables; it usually happens with potatoes, cakes, cookies, and the like. Eventually, too many of those carbohydrate foods are reintroduced. Your body goes out of ketosis (the process of burning fat for fuel), insulin is stimulated, and hunger comes back with a vengeance. Those refined-carbohydrate foods stimulate your desire for more carbohydrate foods and you lose control. Because you've never learned to control those foods in your diet, you gain back your weight (and often more).

People on low-carb diets eat excessive amounts of protein and fat to make up for the missing carbohydrate. The excess protein in your diet must be converted to glucose to provide energy for your muscles and brain. The byproducts of that conversion have to be excreted through your kidneys. If you have kidney disease or are at risk for kidney disease, this can be a problem for you.

To evaluate your own lifestyle and health risks to determine if a lower-carbohydrate diet may be good for you, turn to Chapter 4.

Getting Back to Basics: The Whole Foods Eating Plan

Very-low-carb diets, allowing no more than 15 to 30 grams of total carbohydrate per day, restrict many healthy foods and do not represent balanced lifetime nutrition. However, *moderate* restriction of carbohydrates — below the 60 percent recommended by the USDA, but not to the extreme — can produce positive benefits in many individuals.

Not all carbohydrates are created equally. Certain types of carbohydrates can keep you satisfied longer, and eating a variety of foods keeps you interested in the diet. So which carbs are good and which are bad, and how can you tell the difference? It all depends on the glycemic load of the food. Check out Chapter 3 and Appendix B for more information on glycemic load.

Looking at the changes in food intake and the increase in obesity in the past 20 to 30 years, it's pretty obvious that Americans have gotten away from eating basic whole foods. Much of what we eat is processed, refined, or somehow changed from its original form. Our intake of fruits, vegetables, whole grains, lean protein sources, and good fats is severely lacking.

Introducing the plan

The Whole Foods Eating Plan I've created is designed to help you get back to eating basic healthy foods in a satisfying way. The plan shows you how to lower you total carbohydrate intake in a safe and satisfying way. It shows you how to replace the refined sugars and flour products in your diet with whole, unprocessed fruits and vegetables. You'll discover how to eat quality lean proteins and protective fats. Your appetite needs will be met naturally, and you will not be hungry. Your body will thrive on the nutrients you're feeding it rather than wilting on empty calories. You'll naturally start to lose your surplus fat and your health and energy will soar.

The Whole Foods Eating Plan consists of the following:

- ✔ Vegetables and whole fruits
- ✔ Lean protein, fish, and poultry
- ✔ Low-fat cheese, very low-fat milk, and yogurt

✔ Moderate amounts of fat, especially monounsaturated and polyunsaturated fats such as avocados, olives, olive oil, peanut oil, canola oil, flaxseed oil, and sesame seeds; and nuts and seeds

✔ Whole grains, pasta, and starchy vegetables such as potatoes, corn, and legumes

Sugar, white flour, and other refined grains are limited on the Whole Foods Eating Plan, as are fried foods and processed snack foods.

On the plan, foods are divided into three categories:

✔ **Green Light foods:** The green light means go, go, go. You can move around *freely* in this section and eat as much as you want of Green Light foods.

✔ **Yellow Light foods:** Yellow means slow down and be cautious. Don't let Yellow Light foods get out of control.

✔ **Red Light:** There are no foods in the Red Light category. Red simply means, "Stop and think! You're about to exceed the limit." You can occasionally substitute a sweet-treat for a Yellow Light food. But you must be cautious in doing this and stop before you exceed your limit.

Green Light foods

Eat and drink as many of these foods as you need to satisfy your hunger. Green Light foods include lean meat, fish, poultry, eggs, low-fat cheese, low-fat cottage cheese, salads, non-starchy vegetables, and fresh whole fruits.

For a full list of Green Light foods, check out Chapter 5. You'll also find a great shopping list in Appendix C — don't miss it!

Yellow Light foods

The yellow light is the control feature of the Whole Foods Eating Plan. It allows for your weight loss and lowers your triglycerides and blood sugar if they're elevated. You're allowed five carbohydrate choices per day from the Yellow Light group. A carbohydrate choice is a food that supplies 15 grams of total carbohydrate per serving. (Green Light foods don't count toward this number.) Your five carb choices should ideally be whole grains, beans, or starchy vegetables, but they could be a piece of cake or candy, or a cookie. (Everyone needs a sweet now and then.)

Examples of Yellow Light carb choices include the following:

✔ One slice of regular bread

✔ ½ cup pasta or cereal

✔ ½ cup potatoes, beans, or corn

✔ One serving (15 grams carbohydrate) chips, cookies, cake, or candy

Check out Chapter 6 for the real deal on using your carb choices each day.

Dairy foods and fats

In addition to the five carbohydrate choices, you're allowed the following every day:

- ✔ Two to three servings from the dairy group, which includes skim or low-fat milk, and low-fat yogurt. The carbohydrate in these foods is not counted.

- ✔ Six monounsaturated or polyunsaturated fat choices like avocados, almonds, cashews, peanuts, olives, canola oil, olive oil, or peanut oil; or polyunsaturated fats such as tub or squeeze margarine, reduced-fat mayonnaise, Miracle Whip, salad dressing, corn oil, safflower oil, soybean oil, or sunflower or pumpkin seeds.

For the full scoop on fats, take a look at Chapter 8. Track down the dairy story in Chapter 7.

Red Light foods

Just like on the roadway, the red light means "stop" on the Whole Foods Eating Plan. And stopping is what you should do when you're faced with breads, cookies, cakes, pastries, cereals, gravies, thickened soups, sugar, syrup, chocolate, or soda pop that can cause you to exceed your carbohydrate limit.

No food is absolutely forbidden on the Whole Foods Eating Plan. You just want to make sure that most of the time your five carbohydrate choices per day come from legumes, whole grains, and starchy vegetables in the Yellow Light category. But, if you must have a treat, you can trade it for an equivalent amount of Yellow Light food.

Knowing who can benefit from the plan

If any of the following describes you, you'll benefit from the Whole Foods Eating Plan:

- ✔ You've tried other weight-loss plans and have been unsuccessful.

- ✔ You're overweight or obese (use the BMI table in Appendix A to determine your status).

- ✔ You have or are at risk of developing type 2 diabetes or insulin resistance.

- ✔ You have high triglyceride concentrations in your blood.

- ✔ You have borderline or high blood pressure.

Check out Chapter 4 to determine if lower-carb eating is for you.

Chapter 3

All Carbs Are Not Created Equal: Looking at the Differences

*W*here is carbohydrate? It's in sugar, bread, potatoes, cereal, pasta, beans, chips, cookies, cake, soft drinks, fruit, vegetables, and dairy. It's even a substance in your blood that your body depends on for fuel. Carbohydrate is everywhere except in meats and animal fats, and most of it is pretty tasty. Carbohydrate as a nutrient source is an important part of a healthy diet. To restrict all dietary intake of carbohydrate, the way some low-carb diets prescribe, regardless of its food source is short-sighted. Dismissing fruits, vegetables, whole grains, and beans simply because they contain carbohydrates could be disastrous to your health, in both the short run and the long run.

The intake of refined carbohydrate foods (foods that have been stripped of their nutritional value during processing), yielding little nutritive value except calories, has overwhelmed our sedentary nation. (For more on this situation, take a look at Chapter 2.) Children and athletes can consume larger amounts of starches and sugars with less harm than can relatively inactive people; but many people tend to eat a greater amount of these kinds of carbohydrates than they can handle. So, before you start to lower your carbohydrate intake, you need to get a sense of the various forms and functions of carbohydrates. This will help you decide which ones to keep and which ones to control.

All dietary carbohydrates, from starch to table sugar, can be converted into glucose to be used as fuel for the body, especially the brain. How active you are governs your need for this fuel. So if you're not very active and all your body's reserved carbohydrate fuel is full, you'll store the surplus as fat.

Understanding Carbohydrates

The primary role of carbohydrates in human nutrition is to supply an indispensable commodity — energy. When carbohydrates yield energy at the rate of 4 calories per gram, they spare proteins from being used for energy so that proteins can do the building and repairing of body tissues that they are uniquely suited for. Without sufficient carbohydrate, your body will burn its protein for fuel. Carbohydrates appear in virtually all plant foods and in only one food taken from animals — namely, milk.

The sugar connection

Carbohydrates come in three main sizes: sugars whose atoms are arranged in a single ring (monosaccharides); sugars made from pairs of rings (disaccharides); and long chains of single-ring carbohydrates (polysaccharides). The monosaccharides and disaccharides are known as *simple carbohydrates;* the polysaccharides are known as *complex carbohydrates.* Your body almost invariably converts carbohydrates, whatever form they come in (except dietary fibers), to its own energy source, commonly referred to as *blood sugar.*

What carbs give you beyond nutrition

Six essential nutrients are necessary for good health and for life: protein, carbohydrate, fat, vitamins, minerals, and water. Only protein, carbohydrate, and fat provide energy in the form of calories. Your body needs all these nutrients in order to stay alive. Scientists are learning, however, that there are *other* components that are essential for *good health.* These components don't yield energy either (in other words, they don't have calories), but their role in disease prevention is vital. I cover these non-nutrient components in the following sections.

Fiber

Dietary fiber is found in plant foods and is mainly the fiber component of a plant's cell walls, which aren't digested by the enzymes in your intestinal tract and, therefore, don't provide you with any energy. There are two types of dietary fiber: soluble and insoluble.

As with anything in nutrition, you need a balance of both types of fiber. Soluble fiber helps to lower your LDL ("bad") cholesterol and lowers your rate of glucose absorption. Insoluble fiber helps to soften your stool and lowers your risk of some kinds of cancer. Each type of fiber performs a distinct function and is necessary for good health. (For specifics on working more fiber into your diet, sneak a peek at Chapter 6.)

Traditionally, soluble fiber got the credit for lowering cholesterol, while improvement of bowel regularity was attributed to insoluble fiber. The truth is that both fiber sources improve regularity and lower blood cholesterol.

Phytochemicals

Phytochemicals are compounds that exist naturally in all plant foods (*phyto* comes from the Greek word for "plant"). There are hundreds of thousands of phytochemicals (or *plant chemicals*) in the foods you eat. An apple alone has over 380 kinds of phytochemicals! Carbohydrate foods such as fruits, vegetables, grains, legumes, seeds, licorice root, soy, and green tea all contain these plant chemicals. Phytochemicals are best supplied from fruits and vegetables — not from supplements.

Phytochemicals contain protective, disease-preventing compounds. More than 900 different phytochemicals have been identified as components of food, and many more phytochemicals continue to be discovered every day. Just one serving of vegetables gives you about 100 different phytochemicals!

Think of *phyto* as "fight-o." Every mouthful puts disease fighters in your body. Phytochemicals occur to protect the plant from disease and destruction and continue to protect the humans who eat the plants.

Phytochemicals are associated with the prevention and/or treatment of at least four of the leading causes of death in the United States — cancer, diabetes, cardiovascular disease, and hypertension. They are involved in many processes including those that help prevent cell damage, prevent cancer cell replication, and decrease cholesterol levels.

A sugar by any other name would probably still end in *-ose*

There are six sugars that are most important to nutrition, and they all end in the suffix *-ose*. Originally from the Greek *glykys,* meaning "sweet" and *gleukos,* meaning "sweet wine," the French used the word *glucose* to describe the first discovered simple sugar. Since that time, with each sugar discovery, scientists have continued in the tradition of giving each sugar a name ending with *-ose*. (Think glucose, fructose, galactose, maltose, lactose, and sucrose.) Bottom line: If you see a food label with a listing for something that you don't recognize, and it ends in *-ose,* odds are it's a sugar.

Here's a quick list of a few noteworthy phytochemicals and their sources in carbohydrate foods.

Phytochemical	*Sources*
Allyl sulfides	Garlic, onions, leeks, and chives
Capsaicin	Hot peppers
Carotenoids	Dark green and yellow fruits and vegetables
Coumarins	Citrus fruit, tomatoes
Ellagic acid, phenols	Grapes, berries, cherries, apples, cantaloupe, watermelon
Flavonoids	Citrus fruit, tomatoes, berries, peppers, carrots
Genistein	Beans, peas, lentils
Indoles	Broccoli, cabbage
Isoflavones	Soybeans, dried beans
Lignans	Flaxseed, barley, wheat
Lutein, zeaxanthin	Spinach, kale, collard greens, romaine lettuce, leeks, peas
Lycopene	Tomatoes, red peppers, red grapefruit
Saponins	Soybeans, dried beans
Phytic acid	Whole grains (barley, corn, oats, rye, wheat)

Discovering How Carbs Affect Your Blood Sugar Levels

The glycemic index measures the effects of equal quantities of different carbohydrates on blood glucose levels. Introduced over 20 years ago, the glycemic index challenged traditional thinking about carbohydrate effects on blood sugar. Traditional theory stated that simple carbohydrates, such as orange juice, raised blood glucose levels quickly, while complex carbs, such as crackers, raised blood glucose levels more slowly. However, glycemic index values showed some simple carbohydrates to raise blood glucose slowly and some complex carbohydrates to raise blood glucose quickly.

The *glycemic load* is a measurement that is calculated from the glycemic index and is used to evaluate the glucose response in a normal serving of a particular food. The formula is the glycemic index multiplied by the number of grams of carbohydrate in a serving, divided by 100. Don't worry about the mathematical formulas: Appendix B of this book lists more information on the glycemic index and glycemic load of foods. You can use glycemic load to evaluate the kinds of foods in your diet. If it appears that most of your foods are on the high glycemic load level and those foods are low in nutritive factors, then exchanging some of those high glycemic choices for low glycemic choices would be a good idea. If most of your foods fall into the low glycemic category, then chances are you're eating a very healthy diet.

Carbohydrate foods that are low in glycemic load seem to increase satiety and maintain consistent blood glucose and insulin levels. Non-starchy vegetables, fruits, legumes, and high-fiber whole-grain products tend to have a low glycemic load. These foods have a proven record of health benefits such as lower risk of heart disease and cancer and less gastrointestinal diseases and are a component of any reasonable diet. Such slowly absorbed carbohydrates can contribute greatly to overall health, satiety, and weight loss.

Most refined and processed carbs are high in glycemic load and may result in hunger soon after their rapid digestion. Refined and processed carbs such as those found in cookies, crackers, white bread, and white rice have a high glycemic load; their easy digestion causes a rapid elevation in blood glucose and insulin levels. After a couple of hours, the blood glucose levels quickly decline, resulting in cravings for more food in some people. This phenomenon may have led to the coining of the phrase *carbohydrate addiction*.

You don't have to totally avoid high-glycemic-load foods. You can eat some high-glycemic foods in the presence of low-glycemic foods and the effect on your blood sugar would not be as great as it would be with high-glycemic foods alone. What you need to be aware of is the percentage of high-glycemic-load foods to low-glycemic-load foods. Try to include more low-glycemic-load foods in your diet than high. See Appendix B for more information on glycemic load and glycemic index.

Insulin effects

Insulin follows glucose in the glycemic index response. In other words, as glucose increases, so does insulin. Insulin works to maintain your body's normal blood glucose levels. Some scientists argue that refined carbohydrates like white sugar, white rice, and processed cereals raise blood glucose rapidly, causing an outpouring of insulin. This excess insulin can drop blood glucose levels too rapidly. This sudden drop in blood glucose stimulates hunger and overeating. On the other hand, unrefined carbohydrates such as whole wheat, brown rice, bran cereals, and fruits and vegetables are digested more slowly and contain dietary fiber. These foods raise blood glucose levels slowly without overstimulating insulin, resulting in more-stable blood glucose levels and better appetite control.

Reducing the refined and processed carbohydrates in your diet and tailoring meal plans to your individual needs are safe practices that can have positive effects on your health and well-being. The challenge, as with any healthy modification, is staying motivated to adopt the regimen as a permanent lifestyle change.

Building the Pyramids One Brick at a Time

The USDA Food Guide Pyramid has been around since 1992, and most people know what it is. Versions of the pyramid have been developed for specific age groups such as kids and the elderly, different ethnic groups, and different geographic areas, but they all use a similar organization of foods. Many other pyramids have been proposed to replace the USDA Food Guide Pyramid, such as the Mediterranean Diet Pyramid, the Asian Diet Pyramid, and the Latin American Diet Pyramid. These pyramids emphasize the foods of a particular culture and don't necessarily use the same organization of foods as the USDA Food Guide Pyramid. The Food Guide Pyramid was designed to promote a healthy diet. It includes a variety of whole-grain and fortified refined foods to meet nutrient needs. It was not designed for weight loss.

Unfortunately, even though the Food Guide Pyramid has increased nutrition knowledge, it has not changed eating habits of consumers. The Food Guide Pyramid emphasized moderately lowering fat in the diet and replacing it with bread, cereals, grains, fruits, and vegetables. Fat is a calorie-dense fuel. It provides 9 calories per gram, while carbohydrate and protein each give us 4 calories per gram. Current wisdom would say if you cut out something that gives 9 calories and replace it with something that gives 4 calories, you'll reduce your total calorie intake. Sounds reasonable, right? Take away high-fat foods and replace them with fruits, vegetables, and whole grains. Unfortunately, along with the reduced-fat message came fat-free cookies, cakes, chips, snacks, and desserts. Fat tastes good, so to trick our taste buds into thinking that fat-free foods tasted good, manufacturers loaded it with sugar. So, they didn't just replace a fat gram with a carbohydrate gram in an even swap; they replaced the fat with double, triple, quadruple the carbohydrate!

I favor the Low-Glycemic-Index Pyramid proposed by Dr. David S. Ludwig of Children's Hospital in Boston (see Figure 3-1). The Low-Glycemic-Index Pyramid is designed to prevent and treat obesity. A number of research studies suggest that diets designed to lower the insulin response to ingested carbohydrate (such as a low-glycemic-index diet) may improve utilization of stored energy (body fat), decrease hunger, and promote weight loss. The Low-Glycemic-Index Pyramid demonstrates that such a diet would have as its base abundant quantities of low-glycemic vegetables and fruits, moderate amounts of protein, legumes, reduced-fat dairy, and healthful fats, and an emphasis of whole grains over refined-grain products, potatoes, and concentrated sugars.

Following any diet that doesn't allow you to get the minimum requirements of key nutritional benchmarks, including fiber, calcium, fat, protein, and carbohydrate can have disastrous long-term health complications. Always seek input from your healthcare provider before altering your diet or beginning an exercise program.

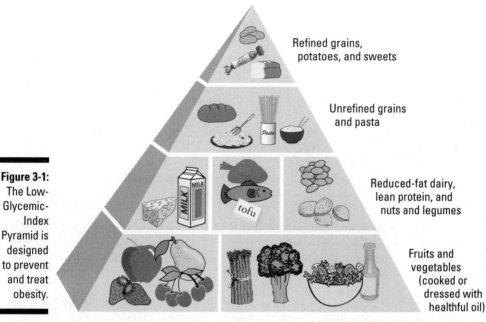

Courtesy of Dr. David S. Ludwig and the Journal of Nutrition

Figure 3-1:
The Low-Glycemic-Index Pyramid is designed to prevent and treat obesity.

Several immediate side effects can occur with a carbohydrate intake of only 20 to 30 grams. Here's a quick list of a few of the most common ones:

✔ **Constipation:** Severe carbohydrate restriction eliminates fruit, vegetables, and grains. The resulting low fiber intake can lead to constipation and gastrointestinal problems.

✔ **Dehydration and low blood pressure:** This results from the excessive water loss in the early stages of the diet.

✔ **Dizziness and fainting:** This can result from low blood pressure due to the dehydration. It's often felt when standing up too quickly.

✔ **Nausea and fatigue:** Both are often associated with ketosis (burning fat for fuel) and low blood-sugar levels.

✔ **Halitosis:** Halitosis is bad breath. It's also associated with an excess amount of ketones (a byproduct of burning fat for fuel) in your body. This occurs when someone is in *ketosis* (the process of burning fat). It has been described as smelling like a cross between nail polish and overripe pineapple. (Just the kind of thing you're striving for, right?)

✔ **Ketosis:** Ketosis is a condition resulting from switching from using carbs to fat as the primary energy source. As your body metabolizes fat, it gives off ketones; excess ketones show up in your urine. Although ketosis is your body's natural backup survival system, when it occurs over an extended period of time, it can cause light-headedness and fogginess. In some medical conditions, prolonged ketosis can cause coma and even death. It is not normal to be in ketosis continually and the long-term safety of this condition is unknown. Ketosis is definitely not good for children.

✔ **Short-term weight loss:** Initial weight loss is due to water loss and levels off in about 7 to 14 weeks. Permanent weight loss occurs more slowly and only if you stay on the diet. When you stop following a low-carb diet and you return to normal eating, the weight usually returns.

Possible *long-term* effects of a very-low-carb diet include the following:

✔ **Loss of muscle mass:** It is essential for your body to have a source of glucose. In diets with too low a restriction in carbohydrate (below 130 grams), your body starts to metabolize the protein in muscle tissue in order to get carbohydrate. This will eventually weaken your body.

✔ **Increased workload on your kidneys:** Very-low-carbohydrate diets are associated with excess protein and fat intake. High protein intake puts an added burden on the kidneys and liver. If you have diabetes, you already have an increased risk of kidney disease, so be sure to check with your physician before following a high-protein diet. If you already have kidney disease, then a low-carb diet is definitely *not* for you.

✔ **Kidney stones and gout:** A high protein, ketosis-inducing diet, can lead to high uric acid levels in the blood, increasing the risk of kidney stones and gout.

✔ **Increased risk of heart disease:** Diets very low in carbohydrate are usually high in saturated fat and high in animal protein. High saturated fat increases the risk of heart disease and some forms of cancer.

✔ **Increased risk of some cancers:** The risk of many cancers is likely to be increased when most fruits, vegetables, whole grains, and beans are eliminated from the diet.

✔ **Osteoporosis:** High animal protein intake combined with the ketosis from a very low carbohydrate intake is thought to draw calcium from the bones, leading to calcium depletion and increasing the risk of osteoporosis and hip fractures. Also, rapid weight loss can accelerate bone deterioration and cause osteoporosis.

✔ **Vitamin and mineral deficiencies:** When entire food groups are eliminated from a diet, such as fruits, vegetables, grains, and dairy, vitamin and mineral deficiencies can occur. High-protein, low-carbohydrate diets usually lack several vitamins and minerals such as vitamins A, C, D, the B vitamins, antioxidants that can slow the effects of aging, and calcium.

None of these complications should occur on the Whole Foods Eating Plan. On the Whole Foods Eating Plan, you're allowed five carbohydrate choices per day, because this is an amount that will allow for a healthy 1 to 2 pounds of weight loss per week. Carbohydrate from fruits and vegetables is not restricted because fruits and vegetables are so essential to good health and disease prevention.

Chapter 4

Determining Whether Low-Carb Eating Is Right for You

In This Chapter

▶ Assessing your personal health history and risks

▶ Looking at your own diet and lifestyle

Not every diet is beneficial to every person. Some people are in perfect health and likely also have nearly perfect diets. Others may need very strict limits or restrictions on foods due to allergies or other conditions. Still others with existing health conditions may need to cut out refined sugars but can enjoy artificially or naturally sweetened foods.

So how do you know if a low-carb diet can benefit you personally? One way is to talk with your family doctor or healthcare professional about the plan I outline in this book. But before you do, consider reading this chapter to get your low-carb ducks in a row. You'll likely be a step ahead when you actually do talk to your doctor, because your doctor will probably want you to complete some version of this assessment.

This chapter is not intended to diagnose your health problems. Its only intent is to make you aware of your risk factors. Healthy adults should have complete physical exams at least every five years beginning at age 20. Check with your family doctor to find out what is appropriate for you.

What's Your Story? Assessing Your Personal Health Risks

People metabolize carbohydrates in different ways. Some carbohydrates are beneficial to your health and others can actually be harmful to your health, depending on your own health history. Before you make a change in your diet, you need to take a look at yourself, your family, and your lifestyle.

Grab a pencil to record the information on your history. And if you haven't seen your family doctor in a while, call and make an appointment to discuss the plan with him or her.

Knowing your BMI, blood glucose (sugar) level, total cholesterol level, HDL cholesterol, LDL cholesterol, triglycerides, and blood pressure is important. You'll probably need to take a trip to your family doctor to get much of this information, although you can determine your BMI in Appendix A, and you may be able to get your blood pressure and cholesterol tested in your community. (YMCAs and even some grocery stores often offer inexpensive blood pressure and cholesterol testing from time to time, so check around.)

Playing detective: Uncovering your family medical history

What kinds of diseases or health problems are in your family? Did Grandma have diabetes? Did Uncle Joe have a heart attack in his forties? Is Uncle Joe Grandma's brother? And, how about Mom and Dad? Are they in good health?

If you're like most people, you probably go through life not really thinking about how your family members' health affects you — but I'm here to tell you it does. Your family's health is part of your own personal health history. That's why your doctor asks you to fill out pages and pages of questions about others in your family (and you thought it was just to keep you occupied while you were waiting to finally get in to see the doctor). Your own health destiny rests, at least in part, in your genes. The sooner you know what you face, the better.

Just because you have a family member who had diabetes or died of a heart attack or cancer doesn't necessarily mean you're destined to have diabetes or heart disease or cancer. But knowing your family's health history does let you know if you're at risk for developing those diseases — and it empowers you to do whatever you can to prevent that from happening.

Start by collecting information from your *first-degree relatives*. A first-degree relative is your brother, your sister, your parents, or your children. Record each disease, illness, or surgery each person has had. Especially ask about chronic illness such as diabetes, heart disease, high blood pressure, cancer, and obesity. If one of your first-degree relatives has died, record the person's age at death and what he or she died of and as much information as you can about any diseases, illnesses, or surgeries he or she had. Especially make note of any disease such as heart disease, cancer, or diabetes that occurred at an unusually early age.

After you've collected all the information you can find on your first-degree relatives, move on to your *extended family*. Your extended family includes grandparents, aunts, uncles, and cousins. If possible, trace your family history back at least three or four generations.

The American Medical Association (AMA) can get you started with their online Adult Family History Form (www.ama-assn.org/ama/pub/print/article/2380-2844.html). You can fill out the form online and then print it for your records. You can also e-mail it to family members for their input. However you gather the information, keep it up to date and share it with your physician and family.

After you've gathered information on your family's health, share it with your family doctor. Especially tell your doctor if you discover two first-degree relatives with the same cancer or one first-degree relative under the age of 50 with an illness usually associated with older people, such as cancer or heart disease.

If you are adopted or have no contact with a biological family, then start keeping a record of what you know about yourself for your current or future offspring.

Figuring out how your age is affecting your health

When it comes to your health, you have control over many, many factors. But one factor you can't control is your age. And as you age, you face increased risk of developing certain diseases. So read on to determine what role your age is playing in your health.

If you get a group of 25-year-olds together, chances are you'll have a very healthy group of people. If you get that same group together 35 years later when they're 60 years old, you'll have a very diverse group in terms of their health status. As we age, we reap the benefits or destruction of our lifestyle, genetics, and exposure. We all want to live long, healthy lives. But that doesn't start at 60 — it starts when we're young. If you're older than 25, don't worry: A healthy lifestyle can start today.

Younger adults

You fall into this age bracket if you're a man between the ages of 20 and 35 or a woman between the ages of 20 and 45.

Heart disease is rare in this age bracket except in those with severe risk factors, such as a genetic tendency for high cholesterol or high triglycerides, heavy cigarette smoking, high blood pressure, or diabetes. Even though heart disease is rare in young adults, *atherosclerosis* (hardening of the arteries) is in its early stages and may progress rapidly. Long-term studies show that high blood cholesterol in young adulthood predicts a higher rate of premature heart disease in middle age.

Smoking and your health

If you're a smoker, quitting smoking is the most important step you can take to improve your health. Smoking increases your risk of lung cancer, throat cancer, the lung disease emphysema, heart disease, high blood pressure, ulcers, gum disease, and other conditions. Smoking can cause coughing, poor athletic ability, and sore throats. It can also cause face wrinkles, stained teeth, and dull skin.

Remember: It is *never* too late to quit smoking. Save your money and prolong your life — quit today. Some people fear the weight gain that sometimes comes with quitting smoking, but it's usually no more than 5 pounds and is easily remedied. The smoking is far worse than the weight gain. Your family doctor or healthcare provider can help you decide which smoking cessation method will work best for you.

Middle-aged adults

You fall into this age bracket if you're a man between the ages of 35 and 65 or a woman between the ages of 45 and 75.

Men generally have a higher risk for heart disease than women. Middle-aged men especially have a tendency to gain weight around the waistline (referred to as *abdominal obesity*), which increases their tendency to become resistant to their own insulin (or suffer from a condition called *insulin resistance*). Insulin resistance can impair your ability to handle blood sugar properly, increase your triglycerides, and lower your HDL ("good") cholesterol. These conditions lead to a dramatically increased risk of heart disease. A sizable portion of all heart disease in men occurs in middle age. Exercise and even a moderate weight loss can dramatically improve the condition.

Heart disease is generally delayed in women by 10 to 15 years compared with men. Therefore, most heart disease in women occurs after the age of 65. Heart disease can occur in women younger than 65 if they're heavy smokers, have high blood pressure, have insulin resistance, have diabetes, or if they have a family history of early heart disease.

Older adults

You fall into this age bracket if you're a man over the age of 65 or a woman over the age of 75.

Most new heart disease events and most heart attack deaths occur in older adults. High blood cholesterol — especially high LDL (or "bad") cholesterol — increases the risk for heart disease in older adults.

Your chances of developing high blood pressure increase with age. Information from the long-running Framingham Heart Study shows that a 55-year-old with normal blood pressure today has a 90 percent chance of developing high blood pressure in the next 25 years.

Looking at your body mass index

The *body mass index* (BMI) is being used as an assessment of body size. In the past, height and weight tables developed by insurance companies classified weights by frame size (small, medium, or large), with one table for men and one for women. The body mass index looks at what people weigh and classifies their weight by degree of medical risk. The BMI is a close measurement of body fat in most people. The same table is used for men and women.

Figuring out your BMI

You can determine your body mass index by using the table in Appendix A. Or you can calculate your body mass index as follows:

1. **Multiply your weight (in pounds) times 703.**

2. **Multiply your height (in inches) times itself.**

3. **Take the number you got in Step 1 and divide it by the number you got in Step 2.**

   The result is your BMI.

For example, let's say you're 5 feet 8 inches tall and you weigh 175 pounds. You would multiply 175×703 to get 123,025. Then you take your height in inches (68 inches) and multiply it times itself (68×68) to get 4,624. Then $123,025 \div 4,624 = 26.6$.

You use the same calculation to figure the BMI for a child over two years of age, but the result isn't interpreted the same as in Table 4-1. Check with your family doctor or pediatrician for the correct interpretation of a child's BMI.

A BMI of 20 to 24.9 is considered a healthy weight. A BMI of 25 to 29.9 is considered overweight, but not obese. And a BMI of 30 or greater is obesity. Refer to Table 4-1 to determine your medical risk based on your BMI.

Get moving: Physical activity and age

You never outgrow your need for physical activity. As you age, you need to be even more dedicated to being active. Normal aging results in a gradual decline in heart and lung function, nerve function, and muscle and bone strength. Being active improves your heart and lungs and allows you to do more work without feeling tired. Physically active older adults have faster reaction times, better balance, and better hand-eye coordination for performing manual tasks. Physical activity can reduce the number of fractures in older adults as well.

Table 4-1	Your Medical Risk Based on Your BMI	
BMI	*Degree of Obesity*	*Degree of Medical Risk*
20 to 24.9	None	None
25 to 29.9	Mild	Low
30 to 34.9	Moderate	Moderate
35 to 40	High	High
Greater than 40	Severe	Severe

In Table 4-1, medical risk is determined just by your weight. You may have an increased medical risk due to other conditions, such as high cholesterol, high blood pressure, diabetes, or some other condition.

Recognizing the limitations of the BMI

Because your BMI is based solely on weight and height, it may overestimate body fat in athletes and others who have a lot of muscle. If this applies to you, you'll need a measure of your body-fat percentage. (Most gyms and fitness centers have facilities and trained personnel to complete these tests.)

On the other hand, BMI may underestimate body fat in older people or others who have lost muscle. So use the BMI as a helpful tool, but realize that its readings and scores are not absolute.

Improving your BMI score

If your number is 30 or above, don't make the mistake of thinking you have to reach the 20 to 25 range before you'll see a benefit to your health. Research shows that if you reduce your weight by 10 percent or even lower your BMI number by 2 points, you'll significantly improve many health factors such as blood glucose, triglycerides, cholesterol, and blood pressure. Give yourself six months to lose 10 percent of your body weight.

If you aren't overweight or obese, but health problems run in your family, keeping your weight steady is important. If you have family members with weight-related health problems, you're more likely to develop them yourself. Talk to your physician if you aren't sure of your risk. Developing a regular habit of physical exercise and eating a healthy diet is the best way to prevent weight gain.

Identifying your diabetes risk

People who have diabetes have a blood glucose level (often called blood sugar level) that is too high. Everyone's blood has some glucose in it because our bodies need it for energy. But too much glucose in the blood isn't good for your health.

There are three main kinds of diabetes:

- ✔ **Type 1 diabetes:** Formerly called juvenile diabetes or insulin-dependent diabetes, type 1 diabetes is usually diagnosed in children, teenagers, or young adults. In this form of diabetes, the body can no longer make insulin. Treatment for type 1 diabetes includes taking insulin shots or using an insulin pump, making wise food choices, exercising regularly, and controlling blood pressure and cholesterol.

- ✔ **Type 2 diabetes:** Formerly called adult-onset or non-insulin-dependent diabetes, this is the most common form of diabetes. People can develop type 2 diabetes at any age — even during childhood. In type 2 diabetes, the body either doesn't make enough insulin or the body can't properly use the insulin it does make; this condition is called *insulin resistance*. Being overweight increases your chances of developing type 2 diabetes. Treatment includes using diabetes medications and sometimes insulin, making wise food choices, exercising regularly, and controlling blood pressure and cholesterol.

- ✔ **Gestational diabetes:** Some women develop gestational diabetes in the late stages of pregnancy. This form of diabetes usually goes away after the baby is born. However, a woman who has had gestational diabetes has a greater chance of developing type 2 diabetes later in life.

Of the more than 17 million Americans with diabetes, most of them have type 2 diabetes, the most common form of the disease. It is estimated that nearly one-third of these people are not even aware they have the disease. One reason is that for a long time, there may not be any warning signs or symptoms. Sometimes the diagnosis may be made only after a serious complication occurs.

Type 2 diabetes is an inherited disease. If you have several family members with the disease, you should be checked for the disease regularly by your physician.

Even though there are different types of diabetes, the signs and symptoms are the same:

- ✔ Extreme thirst

- ✔ Frequent urination

- ✔ Extreme hunger or unusual tiredness

- ✔ Unexplained weight loss

- ✔ Frequent irritability

- ✔ Blurry vision

> ✔ Cuts or sores that heal slowly
>
> ✔ Unexplained loss of feeling or tingling in your feet or hands
>
> ✔ Frequent skin, gum, or bladder infections
>
> ✔ Frequent yeast infections

If you have one sign or symptom, that doesn't mean you have diabetes. But you should start to be concerned if you have several symptoms. A checkup with your doctor now could start you on treatment to help prevent or reduce the heart, eye, kidney, nerve, and other serious complications diabetes can cause.

Recognizing the silent syndrome

A key development in the treatment of diabetes has been a growing understanding of one of its major underlying causes: insulin resistance (also called Syndrome X or Metabolic Syndrome). Our understanding of insulin resistance has resulted in medical treatment options that weren't available even a few years ago.

Insulin resistance occurs when the body fails to respond properly to the insulin it already produces. It is an underlying cluster of symptoms that often precedes the diagnosis of type 2 diabetes. Many people at risk for diabetes do not know what insulin resistance is or even realize that they have signs of diabetes development.

A family history of diabetes, being overweight or obese, and physical inactivity increase your chances of developing insulin resistance. Certain ethnic groups, such as Hispanics, African Americans, and Native Americans, are twice as likely as Caucasians to develop insulin resistance and diabetes. Insulin resistance is associated with an increased risk of heart disease and stroke.

There is no simple test for insulin resistance. However, it's usually marked by a group of characteristics. The presence of three or more characteristics can result in a diagnosis of insulin resistance or metabolic syndrome. The characteristics of insulin resistance syndrome are

> ✔ Abdominal obesity (a waist measuring over 35 inches in women or over 40 inches in men)
>
> ✔ Fasting glucose level of 110 mg/dl or greater
>
> ✔ Triglycerides of 150 mg/dl or greater
>
> ✔ HDL cholesterol less than 50 mg/dl in women or less than 40 mg/dl in men
>
> ✔ Blood pressure of 130/85 or greater

Understanding lipids

Lipid is another name for fat, so blood lipids are fats in your blood. Your doctor can create a *profile* (a breakdown of the different types of fat in your blood) of your lipids to help determine the type of heart disease you are at risk for (if any) and also to help determine the dietary approach to best lower your lipids.

When your doctor or healthcare provider checks your lipids, you're likely to get a list of numbers in each of the following categories:

- **Total cholesterol:** This is a measurement of your total blood fats. This includes the sum of the HDL, LDL, and VLDL cholesterol components.

- **High-density lipoprotein (HDL) cholesterol:** This is commonly called "good" cholesterol because it carries excess cholesterol back to the liver, which processes and excretes the cholesterol. You want this number to be *greater* than 40 mg/dl.

- **Low-density lipoprotein (LDL) cholesterol:** This is commonly called "bad" cholesterol because high levels are linked to increased risk for heart disease. Ideally, you want this number to be *below* 100 mg/dl.

- **Very-low-density lipoprotein (VLDL) cholesterol:** This number is determined by dividing the triglyceride number by 5. VLDL cholesterol can be converted to LDL or "bad" cholesterol.

- **Triglycerides:** Triglycerides are a blood fat that is not only affected by the fat in your diet but is increased by excess calories in the diet and by excess carbohydrate in the diet. It is normal for triglycerides to increase after eating a meal, but they usually fall back to normal in two to three hours. Chronically high triglycerides have recently been linked to heart disease. You want this number to be *below* 150 mg/dl.

Check out Table 4-2 for guidance on what blood lipid levels you should be shooting for.

Table 4-2	Understanding Your Blood Lipid Levels		
Type of Cholesterol	*Desirable*	*Borderline*	*Unacceptable*
Total cholesterol	Less than 200	200 to 239	240 or above
HDL cholesterol	60 or above	40 to 59	Less than 40
LDL cholesterol	Less than 100	100 to 159	160 or above
Triglycerides	Less than 150	150 to 199	200 or above

Spotting early problems with blood pressure

Blood-pressure readings are expressed in two numbers that reflect the pressure on artery walls when the heart contracts. Turn to Table 4-3 for information on what your blood pressure reading means.

Federal health officials recently announced a new category for blood pressure called *prehypertension*. If the top (or systolic) number in your blood pressure reading is between 120 and 139 or if the bottom (or diastolic) number is between 80 and 89, you have prehypertension. Prehypertension is a blood pressure that does not require treatment with medication but still can increase your risk of heart disease and stroke. The new guidelines encourage you to make lifestyle changes such as losing weight, exercising, quitting smoking, or reducing alcohol intake. A dietary approach known as Dietary Approaches to Stop Hypertension (DASH) has been shown to reduce blood pressure. The low-carb eating plan described in this book incorporates the principles of the DASH diet.

Table 4-3	Understanding Your Blood Pressure Reading	
Blood Pressure Classification	**Systolic (Top Number)**	**Diastolic (Bottom Number)**
Normal	Less than 120	Less than 80
Prehypertension	120 to 139	80 to 89
Stage 1 Hypertension	140 to 159	90 to 99
Stage 2 Hypertension	160 or greater	100 or greater

Source: National Heart, Lung, and Blood Institute (NHLBI)

Understanding the relationships between ethnicity and health risks

Certain diseases seem to be more prevalent in some races than others. So with no other issues in your family health history, you still may have risk factors for several diseases just by belonging to a particular ethnic group.

Here's a quick list of some ethnicity-related health concerns. If you belong to any of these groups, pay special attention to the health risks associated with them.

✔ African Americans:

- Have an increased risk for diabetes and insulin resistance
- Are five times more likely than Caucasians to develop kidney disease if diabetic
- Have the highest heart-disease risk and an increased risk for high blood pressure

✔ Asian Americans:

- Have an increased risk for osteoporosis (especially women)

✔ Caucasians:

- Have an increased risk for osteoporosis (especially women)

✔ Latinos:

- Have an increased risk for diabetes and insulin resistance
- Are over six times more likely to develop kidney disease if diabetic

✔ Native Americans:

- Have an increased risk for diabetes and insulin resistance
- Are six times more likely to develop kidney disease if diabetic

Be Honest! Examining Your Current Diet and Lifestyle

After you have an idea of your health status and history, it's time to look at your lifestyle. The good news here is that, unlike your age or your family history, you can make changes to your lifestyle. Some of the risk factors you can change include the foods you eat, how much physical activity you get, whether you smoke, and how much alcohol you drink. If you have family tendencies for diabetes, heart disease, cancer, high blood pressure, and obesity, or if you're starting to show early signs of the conditions yourself, your diet and lifestyle can make those conditions worse or better.

Paying attention to what you eat

An important factor in determining whether a low-carb eating plan is right for you is your willingness to look at your current eating habits. But you can't figure out where you want to go if you don't know where you are.

Recording it

How frequently do chips, crackers, cookies, fast foods, soft drinks, snack foods, cakes, or desserts appear in your food intake? You may not even know the answer to that question. Eating is such a normal daily activity that you may be unaware of what you put in your mouth on a regular basis.

Start keeping a record of everything you eat. Buy a little notebook and keep it handy so you can write down what you eat as soon as you eat. Do this for a week — and be honest (you're only cheating yourself if you aren't). Eat as you normally would. Don't make any changes while keeping the record. If you aren't up to keeping a one-week record, then keep it for a day or two.

Another option is to just sit down and recall what you've eaten in the last 24 hours. Start with your most recent meal and track back for 24 hours. (The only problem with this approach is that you can easily forget about small snack items you ate, like bread or crackers, as well as beverages, all of which should be counted.)

No matter how you do it, develop a picture of your eating pattern. Interestingly, even with all the variety in our food supply, most people eat the same seven to ten meals on a regular basis. So, what does your dietary pattern look like?

Evaluating it

After you have a record of what you've eaten, you need to evaluate how healthy it is. To determine the number of servings you consumed, you'll need to estimate portion sizes. You'll be surprised to see that normal portion sizes are a lot smaller than you think. Here are some examples:

Portion	Approximate Size
½ cup	About the size of a woman's tight fist, or a tennis or billiard ball
1 medium fruit	About the size of a man's tight fist
1 medium potato	About the size of a computer mouse
1 ounce cheese	About the size of your thumb
3 ounces meat	About the size of the palm of a woman's hand or a deck of cards
1 cup	A standard 8-ounce measuring cup

To assess your diet, follow these steps:

1. **Look for the basic foods known to be essential in a healthy diet.**

   Calculate your average daily intake by taking your totals and dividing them by the number of days you kept your food record. For example, if you you've tallied seven fruits over a four-day period, you've consumed an average of 1.75 pieces of fruit each day (7 ÷ 4 = 1.75).

   Use this handy chart to keep track of what you ate.

Foods	Recommended Daily Servings	Number of Servings You Consumed
Fruit	medium piece or ½ cup	2
Vegetables, non-starchy	½ cup	3
Starchy vegetables	½ cup	3
Breads or cereals	1 slice or ½ cup	2
Whole-grain breads or cereals	1 slice or ½ cup	3
Lean meats, poultry, or fish	3 ounces	2
Egg or cheese, low-fat	1 ounce*	1
Milk (skim, ½%, 1%) or yogurt	1 cup	2
Water or other nonsweetened beverage	1 cup	8

* You don't need foods from this category every day.

2. **Look for extra foods that contribute calories but do not contribute significant nutrients.**

   There are no recommended servings in this category so you just need to record your daily intake.

Serving Sizes	*Number You Consumed*
Chips, 1-ounce snack size	_____
Cookies	_____
Dessert, cake, pie, pudding, ½ cup or 1 piece	_____
Ice cream or other frozen desserts, ½ cup	_____
Soft drink, regular, 8 ounces	_____
Meals away from home	_____
Fast-food meals	_____
Hamburger	_____
Cheeseburger	_____
Fried fish or fried chicken	_____
Burritos or tacos	_____
French fries, regular size	_____
Pizza, 1 medium slice	_____
Biscuits, 1 medium	_____
Rolls, 1 medium	_____
Gravy, ¼ cup	_____

3. **Answer the following questions about your food intake:**

   • Did you meet the minimum servings for the basic foods in Step 1?

   • Did your intake of the foods in Step 2 equal or exceed your intake of the foods in Step 1?

   • Can you replace some of your Step 2 choices with Step 1 choices?

   • Are you starting to get the picture of your food habits?

   Step 2 food choices are okay if you're meeting your intake of the basic food groups and if your weight is in the normal range. If you're physically active, you can handle more Step 2 foods than people who aren't very active.

The United States Department of Agriculture's Center for Nutrition Policy and Promotion has an online dietary assessment tool called the Healthy Eating Index (http://147.208.9.33). After entering your food intake for one day (24 hours) you will receive a nutrition analysis including the number of calories you have eaten. You will also receive a score, rating the quality of your food choices.

Determining your level of activity

Being active in today's environment does not come easy. Advances in the modern age have decreased the opportunities for exercise. Television, video games, computerized work centers, and electronic communications have all pulled people indoors and gotten them sitting down. But your body is designed for physical output. You have large muscle groups in your legs, arms, back, chest, and abdomen, and smaller but very important muscles in your organ systems like your heart and lungs. If your muscles don't get the workout they're designed for, your whole body suffers.

Current recommendations for exercise have been increased to one hour of moderate activity five times per week. The new recommendation stems from studies that indicate that people who maintain a healthy weight expend about one hour in moderate activity each day. The good news is that it can be cumulative — you don't have to get in that one hour all at once. The new recommendation means you have to look for opportunities throughout the day to be more active. Taking the stairs, parking farther away, walking to a coworker's desk rather than sending an e-mail, and walking short distances rather than driving a car are just some of the ways to build more exercise into your day. (You can find more on this in Chapter 15.)

Over 60 percent of Americans don't participate in the recommended amount of exercise and about 25 percent of Americans are not physically active at all. Even light activities such as standing or walking around the house are better than no activity at all. If you aren't very active, start gradually and build up.

Look at the following categories of activity and mark the one that comes closest to describing how you spend your week. Unless you're in the active or very active category, plan to up your exercise by one level.

- **Sedentary:** Watching television, driving a car, sitting at work, playing board games, sewing, reading, writing, talking on the phone. No program of regular exercise.

- **Light exercise:** Ironing, dusting, doing laundry, loading/unloading the dishwasher, preparing and cooking food, walking 2 miles per hour for 10 to 20 minutes 3 to 5 times per week.

- **Moderate exercise:** Dancing, gardening, doing carpentry work, mopping/scrubbing, bicycling, jogging or walking at 3 miles per hour for 20 to 40 minutes 3 to 5 times per week.

- **Active:** Heavy work, aerobics, tennis, skating, skiing, racquetball, brisk walking at 4 miles per hour for 30 to 60 minutes 3 to 5 times per week.

- **Very active:** Bicycling 15 miles per hour, running 6 miles per hour, swimming, or participating in martial arts, for 45 to 60 minutes 3 to 5 times per week.

Discovering the effects of stress

Stress is unavoidable, but it can be good or bad. Normal transitions in life like getting married or having a baby bring about stress. A job promotion that calls for a move to a new city brings about stress. Other kinds of stress can bring prolonged responses. An unpleasant coworker or difficult job situation is there every day. You have to manage a decrease in your finances every day. Significant stress events like the death of a spouse or child never fully go away. Stress is part of living.

Alcohol: Moderation is the key

Alcohol is a culturally accepted drug. Many people drink alcohol at some point in their lives. Some only drink during social occasions and others may have an evening glass of wine. Moderate alcohol consumption can reduce your risk of heart disease. However, the benefit is not so great that a non-drinker should consider drinking alcohol. About one-third of those drinking alcohol will develop problems with alcohol. Drinking problems can increase your risk of serious health problems (both physical and behavioral) and accidents or injuries.

If you want to drink alcohol, moderate consumption is considered safe. Moderate drinking is considered two drinks a day for men, and one drink a day for women or lighter-weight men. A drink is 12 ounces of beer, 5 ounces of wine, or 1½ ounces of hard liquor, as shown in the illustration. Be sure to count these beverages in your daily five carbohydrate choices. Each one counts as one carbohydrate choice.

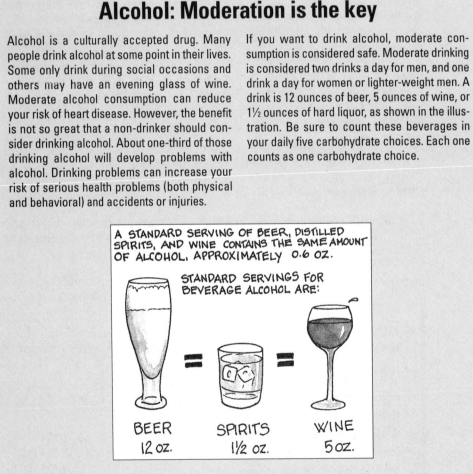

A STANDARD SERVING OF BEER, DISTILLED SPIRITS, AND WINE CONTAINS THE SAME AMOUNT OF ALCOHOL, APPROXIMATELY 0.6 OZ.

STANDARD SERVINGS FOR BEVERAGE ALCOHOL ARE:

BEER 12 oz. = SPIRITS 1½ oz. = WINE 5 oz.

How you deal with the stress is what's important. Some people respond to stress by eating poorly, being physically inactive, smoking, or drinking alcohol. Others criticize their spouses, yell at their kids, and kick their dogs. And some employ the silent treatment — keeping everything bottled up inside when they're about to explode. All these reactions take their toll on your body.

Short-term responses to stress can be a headache, stomachache, diarrhea, constipation, or vomiting. Longer-term responses affect blood pressure and sleeping and increase your risk for depression, heart disease, and susceptibility to colds and infections.

Eating and bingeing just compound the stress. The temporary comfort provided by the food is followed by guilt for overeating. Stress is pent-up energy that needs to be released. When stress comes, step back, take a deep breathe, and go for a walk. Buy yourself some time to relax and decompress.

If your problems with stress are far more serious, talk to a trusted friend, your pastor, your family doctor, or a professional counselor.

Deciding Whether a Low-Carb Diet Can Help

A low-carb diet, especially one like the Whole Foods Eating Plan, can help the following conditions:

- ✔ Overweight (BMI of 25 to 29.9)
- ✔ Obesity (BMI of 30 or greater)
- ✔ Type 2 diabetes
- ✔ Insulin resistance
- ✔ Heart disease
- ✔ High triglycerides
- ✔ Low HDL cholesterol
- ✔ High blood pressure (but only if the low-carb plan allows fruits, vegetables, low-fat dairy, whole grains, nuts, and seeds)
- ✔ Polycystic ovarian syndrome (PCOS), a disease in women associated with insulin resistance

If you suffer from any of the preceding conditions, going the healthy low-carb route may be exactly what your body needs. However, if you have kidney problems, you may want to find another eating plan.

As with any diet plan, be sure to consult your doctor or registered dietitian to determine if this plan is safe for you to follow given your specific health situation. (For the full story on the Whole Foods Eating Plan, check out Part II.)

Part II
Steering Yourself Back to Whole Foods

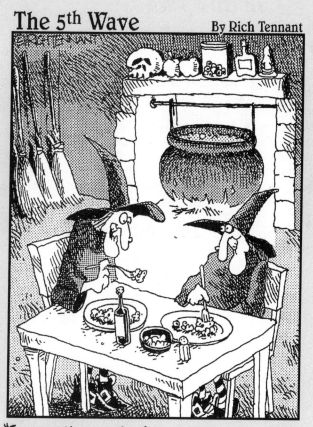

The 5th Wave   By Rich Tennant

"I substitute tofu for eye of newt in all
my recipes now. It has twice the protein
and doesn't wriggle around the cauldron."

In this part . . .

I steer you back to basic, whole, unprocessed foods. You'll travel to the Whole Foods Eating Plan, a reduced-carbohydrate approach that I've developed and used successfully at Texas Tech Medical Center. You can taste the wholesome goodness of the foods from the earth as you travel down the food freeway, paved with fruits and vegetables. You'll choose quality proteins without choosing fat. You'll set your cruise control on carbohydrates, shift into high gear with lean proteins and dairy foods, and fuel up on good fats. Here, I show you how you can navigate the Whole Foods Eating Plan for the rest of your life.

Chapter 5

Taking a Joyride: Falling in Love with Whole Foods

About five years ago, I began to take a look at the fad diets that people found so appealing. Simplicity and the quick weight-loss results they promised were very attractive. But restrictive food choices and the inability to sustain the weight loss round out the fad-diet story. I saw people who were overwhelmed by the modern diet of super-sized fast foods, soft drinks, and salty and fat-free snacks — and their health was suffering. I also saw them struggling to lose weight by following a fad diet.

A friend gave me a fad diet for my collection that had one particularly appealing feature: It allowed you to eat as much as you wanted of certain fruits and vegetables. Other aspects of the diet weren't healthy — like allowing free intake of high-fat meats and dairy items, including bacon, sausage, butter, and whole milk — but I was intrigued by the idea of "free" foods.

Knowing how far the American diet had drifted from the basics of good health, allowing convenient refined and processed foods to replace simple, nutritional food, I used the free-food idea to develop a plan that would turn people back to basic *whole foods* (foods with little processing). Essentially, I let the foods I wanted people to eat become *free foods*. The participants could eat as many of the free foods as they wanted, whenever they wanted, without restrictions. The results of the experiment were encouraging. People not only lost weight but told me how easy following the plan was. They were eating a lot healthier, and they didn't feel deprived!

I originally designed the Whole Foods Eating Plan for weight loss in our clinics at Texas Tech. However, with medical supervision, I've used the plan to benefit people with diabetes, high triglycerides, high blood pressure, and related health problems. The plan helps you control, but doesn't entirely eliminate, the intake of refined sugars and flour, and it encourages you to eat whole, unprocessed foods. You may be surprised to see that the plan contains moderate amounts of starch, protein, and fat. That's because the plan allows your nutrition needs to be supplied *naturally* with healthy foods.

If you hate counting calories and grams, this chapter is definitely for you. Here, I show you the fruits, vegetables, and lean protein that are yours for the taking as free foods. (You can eat free foods in unlimited quantities — they're free because you don't pay for them by counting calories or using food-group choices like you might on another diet plan.) This "food freeway" is the first leg of your journey to your destination of the Whole Foods Eating Plan. The plan is not a quick fix for getting rid of some extra pounds; it's a journey that can steer you back to healthy eating without forcing you to think much about quantities. But don't worry — on this trip, you'll also drop some excess baggage (in the form of unwanted pounds) along the way.

Even if you decide that the Whole Foods Eating Plan isn't for you, you can likely benefit from the information in the chapter and create your own low-carb plan. Removing processed foods, or at least reducing the amount of processed foods, from your diet is a fantastic change to just about anyone's diet. Just knowing which foods are the healthiest for you can help shape your eating in a healthier direction for the rest of your life.

Green-Light Foods: Knowing Which Foods You Can Eat without Thinking Twice

The Whole Foods Eating Plan is paved with fruits, vegetables, and protein foods, such as lean meat, fish, poultry, and low-fat cheeses. I don't want you to be hungry on this eating plan. Instead, I want you to satisfy your hunger with fruits, vegetables, and lean protein foods. I mark each list of free foods in this chapter with a Green Light icon, which means "Go ahead and make your choice."

Green Light foods are the heart and soul of this low-carb diet. You don't have to weigh or measure Green Light foods — you can eat as much as you want whenever you want. Understanding portion sizes is important, of course, and I discuss portions in Chapters 6, 7, and 8. But in this chapter, I help you replace the highly refined carbohydrates in your diet with Green Light foods.

Too good to be true?

When I first started allowing fruits, veggies, and meats to be free, I was often asked if I was afraid people would eat too much of these foods. I did have some concerns when I developed this plan, but here's what I found: Some folks did overindulge in the early stages of the eating plan, but when they realized they weren't restricted on amounts, they would drop back to reasonable portion sizes.

Exploring the Free Carbs: Fruits and Vegetables

Fruits and vegetables are as good as it gets, so don't hold back! You can eat and drink as much of the carbohydrates listed in this section as you need to satisfy your hunger. The fruits and vegetables in this group do contain carbohydrates, but they're low on *glycemic load,* which ranks foods according to how they affect your blood-sugar level. The fruits and vegetables on this list are whole foods, packed with nutrients!

The glycemic load of foods shows how rapidly a food is digested, thus driving up the blood sugar. Insulin, which lowers your blood sugar, is also stimulated. Foods with a high glycemic load cause a spike in your blood-sugar level, and then insulin quickly lowers it. This sudden change in your blood-sugar level can actually *cause* hunger. (Imagine, you could be even hungrier after you eat these foods than you were before!) Foods with a low glycemic load cause a gradual, moderate increase in blood sugar without overstimulating insulin and are more satisfying to your appetite. See Chapter 3 and Appendix B for more details on the glycemic load.

Eat and be merry with as many of the carbohydrates listed in the following sections as you need to satisfy your hunger. And remember, *free* really does mean free. You don't have to weigh or measure these foods.

To make eating fruits and vegetables more convenient, I suggest these strategies:

✔ **Select fruits and vegetables that require little peeling and chopping.** Good options include baby carrots, cherry tomatoes, asparagus, grapes, apples, and broccoli spears.

✔ **Shop the supermarket salad bars.** They offer many favorite raw vegetables and fresh fruits already cleaned and sliced.

✔ **Put fruits that don't need refrigeration where you can see them.** Make a habit of grabbing a few pieces on your way out the door.

✔ **Shop seasonal specials for better prices.**

Making fruit choices — fresh is best

Fruit is the original fast food. Nature has nicely packaged it for easy take-out. When possible, choose fresh, whole, naturally ripe fruit. But if fresh isn't available, you can buy frozen fruit year-round. If you use canned, choose fruit in 100-percent fruit juice instead of sugary syrup. If you have to buy canned fruit in a light syrup, drain it before eating. In most cases, frozen and canned fruits are just as nutritious as fresh. Besides, eating canned and frozen fruits is better than eating no fruit at all!

Bananas are not on the Green Light food list. It's not that I don't want you to eat bananas — you can find them in Chapter 6 on a Yellow Light list signaling caution. Bananas are a very good food and the number-one fruit sold in the United States. However, they're starchier than other fruits, so I count them like bread. People who eat bananas tend to eat a lot of them. So, if I gave bananas a Green Light, some people would only eat bananas and no other fruit! *Remember:* Always eat a variety of fruits.

Wash fruit as soon as you get home from the store (even those with heavy peels like oranges). Then you can grab some directly from the fruit bowl or crisper on your way out. Berries and grapes are the only exceptions; wash them the day you eat them and not before.

Here's a list of the Green Light, or free, fruits. So, go, go, go, and eat them up!

- **Apples, dried:** Dried apples make a great snack food and are easy to transport.

- **Apples, fresh:** It makes no difference what variety of apple you choose. My favorite is Golden Delicious. Availability changes with the seasons, though.

- **Applesauce, unsweetened:** Applesauce isn't just for kids! Grownups love this tart sauce, too.

- **Apricots, dried:** Dried apricots make a nice snack — the dense, sweet-tart apricot taste can be quite addictive.

- **Apricots, fresh:** Apricots are a smooth, sweet summer fruit chock-full of nutritional goodness.

- **Blackberries:** Blackberries are as big as your thumb, purple and black and thick with juice. I remember picking these as a kid while catching June bugs and watching for snakes.

- **Blueberries:** Blueberries are late-summer berries with a very rich taste. They're great sprinkled in a salad!

- **Cantaloupe:** Cantaloupe comes with its own bowl — just cut it in half and scoop out each half with a spoon.

- **Cherries, sweet, canned:** When you buy canned cherries, you're getting two for the price of one — the fruit and the canned juice.

- **Cherries, sweet, fresh:** Go for fresh cherries when possible, and use frozen ones in a pinch. Canned syrupy pie filling is overloaded with sugar and corn starch, so avoid it.

- **Dates:** A few dates are all you need to fill up.

- **Figs, dried:** Dried figs are readily available year-round. The easiest way to chop them is to snip them with scissors.

- **Figs, fresh:** Fresh figs are a healthy fruit that can satisfy a craving for sweetness.

- **Fruit cocktail:** When was the last time you had a serving of this pitch-in dinner specialty?

- **Grapefruit:** America's wake-up fruit, this eye-opener may be rosy-fleshed or white.

- **Grapefruit sections, canned:** Keep canned grapefruit in the pantry, always ready to go.

- **Grapes:** Good nutrition comes in small packages.

- **Honeydew melons:** "Honey, dew try this!" (I couldn't resist.)

TIP

Juices, juices everywhere, but how many drops (or ounces) to drink?

Choose real fruit juice, not fruit drink. Fruit drink is only 10 percent real fruit juice or less — the rest is sugar water! Drink fruit juice instead of sodas or coffee in the car. You can keep 8- to 12-ounce bottles in your refrigerator chilled and ready to go! Or you can by them at gas stations and fast-food chains. If you need a big gulp, combine a 6-ounce juice with a 12-ounce can of *diet* lemon-lime or ginger ale soda.

Give these healthy juices a try:

- **Apple juice/cider:** Apple juice beats a can of soda any time and doesn't take as much to satisfy your hunger.

- **Cranberry juice cocktail, reduced-calorie, light:** Cranberries lessen bladder infections by preventing bacteria from clinging to the inside of the bladder and urinary tract. To avoid too much sugar, always buy the light version of cranberry juice.

- **Fruit juice blends, 100-percent juice:** Fruit-juice blends are a delicious drink of pure juice.

- **Grape juice:** Grape juice is healthy for the heart.

- **Grapefruit juice:** Grapefruit juice makes a great snack between meals.

- **Orange juice:** Make it fresh whenever possible. It's worth the extra effort.

- **Pineapple juice:** You can use pineapple juice to sweeten less-sweet fruits.

- **Prune juice:** This will improve your bowel regularity. Don't be afraid to try it.

TECHNICAL STUFF

Low-calorie sweeteners

Low-calorie sweeteners, sometimes referred to as *artificial sweeteners,* add to foods a taste that is similar to table sugar. These intense sweeteners are generally several hundred to several thousand times sweeter than sugar, however. Most don't contain calories and those that do are used in very small amounts because of their concentrated sweetening power. Thus, they add essentially no calories to foods and beverages. These sweeteners practically eliminate or substantially reduce the calories in some foods and beverages such as carbonated soft drinks, light yogurt, and sugar-free puddings. Low-calorie sweeteners result in a wide range of food choices that can help you manage your intake of calories and carbs. Using these sweeteners may help you in the early stages reducing your carbohydrate intake.

- ✔ **Kiwis:** Don't let the hairy green skin turn you off this exotic little gem — just don't forget to peel it! One kiwi has more vitamin C than ½ cup of orange juice.

- ✔ **Lemons:** You can use lemon to add flavor to any beverage. They're great to keep in the fridge for salad dressings, as a quick flavor for fish, or to give the flavors of your other fruits a twist.

- ✔ **Limes:** Limes are highly underrated in the United States. I use lime to flavor everything from water and diet sodas to anything with cilantro, including salsa. Its crisp, fresh flavor makes just about everything taste better.

- ✔ **Mandarin oranges, canned:** Mandarin oranges are Chinese oranges that are very sweet! Drain them well and add to any dish.

- ✔ **Mangos:** Mango is delicious by itself or paired with other tropical fruits, like papaya. Their flavor is something like a tangy peach.

- ✔ **Nectarines:** Nectarines are a smooth-skinned variety of peach. They taste best at the height of the season (in late June and July).

- ✔ **Oranges:** Oranges are a fall and winter fruit. When eaten raw, none of its precious vitamin C is lost.

- ✔ **Papaya:** You can bake unripe papayas like squash. They contain *papain,* the predominant ingredient in meat tenderizer.

- ✔ **Peaches, canned:** Canned peaches make a quick dessert for any meal.

- ✔ **Peaches, fresh:** Don't let a little peach fuzz keep you away. Peaches are delicious and loaded with nutrients.

- ✔ **Pears, canned:** Cut up canned pears and add them to a salad.

- ✔ **Pears, fresh:** You can purchase pears green and they will continue to ripen. They *do* get sweeter as they ripen!

- ✔ **Pineapple, canned:** Always buy canned pineapple in its own juice instead of syrup.

- ✔ **Pineapple, fresh:** Known as a symbol of hospitality in the South, fresh pineapple makes a sweet dessert.

- ✔ **Plums, canned:** Canned plums are a readily available treat.

- ✔ **Plums, fresh:** Plums come from trees found in every continent in the world except Antarctica.

- ✔ **Prunes, dried:** Prunes are dried, small, purplish-black, freestone plums. They're very rich in flavor. You can also find them infused with essence of orange and lemon.

- ✔ **Raisins:** Raisins are just dried grapes. They make a handy snack.

- ✔ **Raspberries:** When they are fully ripe, raspberries' caps detach. Midsummer is their prime season.

- ✔ **Strawberries:** Strawberries are a super food chock-full of health-giving nutrients.

- ✔ **Tangerines:** Tangerines are small, sweet, Chinese oranges. They peel so easily it's as if they have a zipper.

- ✔ **Watermelon:** Watermelon is a summertime treat that can't be beat! Try freezing watermelon juice in ice-cube trays and adding the cubes to drinks.

Go easy on fruit juices! Don't let all your fruit servings come from juice. Try to eat at least one piece of whole fruit every day. But when you do reach for a glass of juice, make it ½ cup to 1 cup of 100-percent fruit juice with no sugar added.

To increase your fruit intake, try these suggestions:

- ✔ Nibble on grapes or raisins.

- ✔ Blend fresh fruit with your morning yogurt. Add a splash of orange juice and crushed ice for a homemade smoothie.

- ✔ Add strawberries or blueberries to your green salad.

- ✔ Try frozen bing cherries for an instant treat.

- ✔ Make your own sorbet or granita with sweet, fresh berries.

Eating your veggies, the nutrition superstars

Vegetables are nutrition superstars! They're low in calories and fat, cholesterol-free, and high in vitamins, minerals, cancer fighters, and heart protection. Veggies are nature's defense mechanism, protecting you against disease — and in the American diet, they're neglected.

Be adventurous and get acquainted with a new vegetable each week. You're in for a pleasant surprise.

You may have these vegetables cooked, raw, canned, frozen, microwaved, steamed, or stir-fried (but not deep-fried, breaded, or creamed), with no limits on amounts:

- **Artichokes:** I don't recommend eating artichokes raw — not even in Texas. Take a look at Figure 5-1 for instructions on cleaning and trimming an artichoke.

- **Artichoke hearts:** Artichoke hearts make delicious salad material.

- **Asparagus:** Asparagus is a special, delicious vegetable, once only available to kings.

- **Bean sprouts:** Bean sprouts are the basis of a good stir-fry.

- **Beans (green, wax, Italian):** Beans are a go-with-anything vegetable.

- **Beets:** Plain or pickled, you can use the tops of beets as greens.

- **Broccoli:** Broccoli is America's favorite vegetable — despite what the first President Bush thinks.

- **Brussels sprouts:** This tiny, green, cabbage-like vegetable is a big defender of good health.

Cleaning an Artichoke

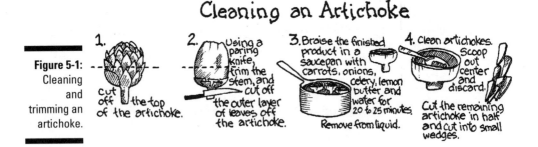

Figure 5-1: Cleaning and trimming an artichoke.

- **Cabbage:** Cabbage is a big cousin to the Brussels sprout. It packs a wallop against cancer and is a nutrition powerhouse.

- **Carrots:** It's true — carrots are good for your eyes.

- **Cauliflower:** The "flower of the cabbage" is a nutritious bouquet.

- **Celery:** Often seen on the relish tray, you can combine celery with anything.

- **Cucumbers:** The cucumbers you find in the supermarket are often waxed, which means you have to peel them before eating. If the skin is not waxed, however, it's edible.

- **Eggplant:** A purple powerhouse of prevention, eggplant should always be eaten cooked.

- **Green onions or scallions:** Green onions are sweetest when the bulbs are thinnest.

- **Greens (collard, kale, mustard, turnip):** Greens are versatile vegetables of many virtues. Vary the way you serve greens, just to shake things up.

- **Kohlrabi:** The knobs of kohlrabi are thickened stems. Kohlrabi is superb in flavor, but unless the plant is young, it's frequently too fibrous in texture to be worth preparing.

- **Leeks:** A cousin to the onion, leeks are good heart medicine and may help prevent cancer. Be sure to soak and wash leeks thoroughly in order to remove dirt and sand deep down in the bulb. Figure 5-2 shows you how to clean and trim leeks.

Cleaning & Trimming Leeks

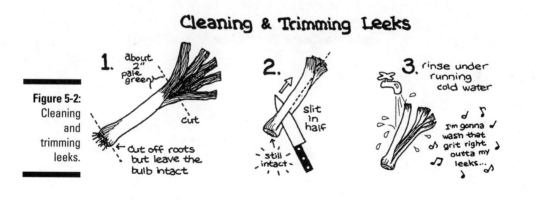

Figure 5-2: Cleaning and trimming leeks.

- **Mushrooms:** Unless you're a mushroom expert, buy your mushrooms in a market. Those nice-looking mushrooms that pop up in your yard after a rain can be deadly.

- **Okra:** When included in stews, okra's gluey sap helps thicken the sauce.

- **Onions:** The old-time cough medicine of onion juice and honey was nothing to sneeze at. The substance in onions that makes you cry also breaks up mucous congestion.

- **Pepper (all varieties):** Sweet or hot, peppers are full of zesty nutrition. Figure 5-3 shows you how to core and seed a bell pepper.

- **Radishes:** Often transformed into a clever garnish, radishes are good to eat.

- **Salad greens (endive, escarole, lettuce, romaine, spinach):** I'm not talking anemic iceberg lettuce here, but dark, leafy greens that are full of compounds to help you resist disease. Use several varieties together in your salad.

- **Salsa and picante sauce:** Salsa adds pizzazz to anything!

- **Sauerkraut:** To retain its full flavor, sauerkraut should be served raw or barely heated through. Cooking makes kraut milder.

- **Snow peas:** Snow peas are excellent in salads, stir-fry, or featured on a veggie platter.

- **Spinach:** Tender young spinach works best in salads, either alone or mixed with other greens. Even a greens-hating child may enjoy spinach in salads.

How to Core and Seed a Pepper

Figure 5-3:
Coring and
seeding bell
pepper.

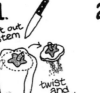

1.
cut out
stem
twist
and
pull
out

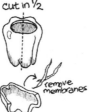

2. cut in ½
remove
membranes

3.
Cut into
lengthwise
strips

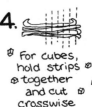

4.
For cubes,
hold strips
together
and cut
crosswise

- **Squash, summer:** Summer squash is delicious raw or cooked.

- **Tomatoes, fresh:** The red color of tomatoes signals the presence of lycopene, a phytochemical that protects against cancer. Look for other tomato varieties in your market as well, including green zebra, yellow teardrop, pear, grape, and cherry. So many choices, so little time!

- **Tomato sauce:** Cooking doesn't destroy lycopene. It actually makes it better. So tomato sauce is a good source of the cancer fighter.

- **Tomato/vegetable juice:** Tomato juice, whether alone or combined with other vegetables juices, makes a great healthy drink — any time, any place.

- **Tomatoes, canned:** Canned tomatoes fill in nicely when fresh tomatoes are out of season.

- **Turnips:** Peel turnips before cooking; the peel gives a bitter flavor to the vegetable.

- **Water chestnuts:** Combine the crunchy, crisp vegetable with other veggies.

- **Watercress:** Watercress adds a distinctive flavor to salads, sandwiches, soups, and vegetables. Never overcook it — it becomes stringy when overcooked.

- **Zucchini:** Zucchini is a versatile green squash — cooked or raw.

Strictly speaking, a tomato is a fruit, not a vegetable (some nonsense about it having internal seeds that can later germinate into fruit berry plants, yada yada yada). But for the purposes of this book, I'm just going to keep it in the vegetable category, where everyone expects it.

To increase your vegetable intake, try these suggestions:

- Pile lettuce, sprouts, and tomatoes on your sandwich.

- Enjoy soup or salad with a variety of vegetables.

- Pack zucchini slices, baby carrots, or celery sticks in your lunch.

- Chop raw veggies and add them to your green salad.

- Steam your own mixed veggie combinations with a variety of seasonings. Vary it by the day (carrots, cauliflower, and snow peas on Monday; zucchini, yellow squash, and red onions on Tuesday; and so on).

- Sautee spinach in a tiny bit of olive oil with garlic for a super quick, warm salad.

Cruciferous cabbage to the rescue!

The term *cruciferous* simply means vegetables in the cabbage family whose leaves form a crucifix or cross. This includes bok choy, broccoli, Brussels sprouts, cabbage, cauliflower, kale, mustard, and turnip greens, among others. Cabbage-family vegetables contain compounds that stop processes in the body that can develop into cancer.

The cabbage-family vegetables are

✔ **Bok choy:** This delicious Chinese cabbage comes in several varieties but is most commonly found in the United States in regular and baby varieties. Baby bok choy, prized for its tender delicate texture, can be cooked whole. The larger variety needs to be cut before cooking. Bok choy greens resemble green leaf lettuce while the white stalks have the crunch of celery without its "strings." Bok choy is an excellent source of vitamin C, calcium, and folic acid; it's great added to stir-fried vegetable dishes and soups.

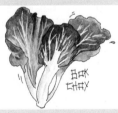

✔ **Broccoli:** Try broccoli sprouts, too, for a punch of nutrition in salads and on sandwiches.

✔ **Brussels sprouts**

✔ **Cabbage:** Choose red cabbage for its abundance of vitamin C. Savoy cabbage has extra beta carotene. And even the common green cabbage can't be beat for its wealth of nutrients.

✔ **Cauliflower**

✔ **Daikon:** This is a jumbo-sized Japanese radish sometimes exceeding 3 feet in length! The size typically used in the kitchen is about the size of a carrot. Though daikon looks like a large white carrot, it tastes kind of like a radish, but hotter.

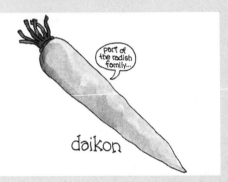

part of the radish family...

daikon

✔ **Kale**

✔ **Kohlrabi:** Sometimes called the "cabbage turnip," this cabbage has a swollen stem, resembling a root. It is crisp and juicy, with a surprising mixture of sweetness, much like an apple, with a slight peppery bite like a radish. Both the leaves and stems can be eaten fresh, steamed, braised, sautéed . . . you name it.

✔ **Mustard greens**

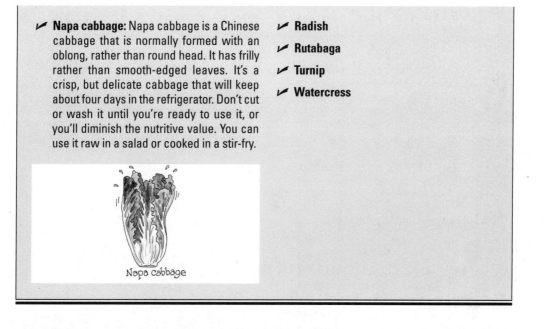

✔ **Napa cabbage:** Napa cabbage is a Chinese cabbage that is normally formed with an oblong, rather than round head. It has frilly rather than smooth-edged leaves. It's a crisp, but delicate cabbage that will keep about four days in the refrigerator. Don't cut or wash it until you're ready to use it, or you'll diminish the nutritive value. You can use it raw in a salad or cooked in a stir-fry.

✔ **Radish**

✔ **Rutabaga**

✔ **Turnip**

✔ **Watercress**

Napa cabbage

Indulging in Free Proteins

Protein is an important part of a healthy diet. Its function is to build and repair body tissues. Proteins from animal sources like meat, fish, dairy, and egg products are valued because their total protein content is high. They're referred to as *complete proteins* because they contain all the essential *amino acids* (the building blocks for constructing and repairing body tissues) required from your diet. However, many animal protein sources are also associated with saturated fat. Saturated fat contributes to heart disease by raising your cholesterol level. Choose animal proteins that are low in saturated fat.

Scientific studies show that in some people replacing some of the carbohydrate in a diet with lean protein lowers triglyceride levels and raises HDL cholesterol levels. That's good, because high triglycerides and low HDL cholesterol have been identified as risk factors for heart disease. Plus, if you eat some protein instead of carbs, you feel satisfied sooner!

Meat and cheese choices

Meat and cheese contain many good nutrients, but the fat in these foods is mostly saturated fat, and you need to limit your intake of saturated fat. Meat and cheese choices should have no more than 5 grams of fat per ounce. In the following sections, the number listed in brackets after each food is the number of grams of fat per ounce. To reduce saturated fat even further, choose the foods with 3 grams of fat per ounce, such as beef sirloin, or 0 to 1 gram of fat per ounce, such as chicken.

Beef

Lean beef is an excellent protein choice. You can eat it several times per week. Choose USDA Choice or Select grades of lean meat. Avoid heavily marbled (high-fat) meats because they're high in saturated fat.

- Corned beef [5 grams of fat per ounce]
- Flank steak [3]
- Ground beef, lean [3]
- Ground beef, regular [5]
- Prime rib [5]
- Roast (rib, chuck, rump) [3]
- Round [3]
- Short ribs [5]
- Sirloin [3]
- Steak (T-bone, porterhouse) [3]
- Tenderloin [3]

Making the grade

Beef grading is conducted by the U.S. Department of Agriculture (USDA). Inspectors grade, or rate, meat based on the amount of *marbling* (flecks of fat within the lean portion of the meat) and the age of the animal. These quality grades are an indication of tenderness, juiciness, and flavor.

The most readily available grades are Prime, Choice, and Select. *Prime* has the most marbling

(and the most fat and flavor). It is produced in limited quantities and usually sold to fine restaurants and specialty meat markets. *Choice* falls between Prime and Select. Of these three, *Select* has the least amount of marbling, making it leaner than, but often not as tender, juicy, and flavorful as, the other two top grades. Most markets today offer a selection of Choice and Select cuts.

Pork

Pork is a lot leaner these days and you can include it in a healthy diet. Prepackaged hams usually have only a fraction of the fat of a whole ham.

- Boston butt [5 grams of fat per ounce]
- Canadian bacon [3]
- Center loin chop [3]
- Cutlet, unbreaded [3]
- Ham (fresh, canned, cured) [3]
- Tenderloin [3]

Lamb

A favorite meat around the world, the leanest cuts of lamb are leg, arm, shank, and loin.

- Chop [3 grams of fat per ounce]
- Leg [3]
- Roast [5]

Veal

Veal is a favorite meat in Italy. All cuts of veal are lean; it's what we tend to do to them — breading, like Veal Parmigiana, thick butter sauces, like Veal Picatta, and so on — that make veal not so healthy.

- Chop, trimmed of visible fat [3 grams of fat per ounce]
- Cutlet (unbreaded) [3]
- Roast [3]

Game

Game meats are leaner than domestic meats. Some wild game, such as venison and rabbit, are very lean. Some exotic "new" meats also low in fat are ostrich, emu, and buffalo.

- Alligator [0–1 gram of fat per ounce]
- Buffalo [0–1]
- Emu [0–1]
- Ostrich [0–1]
- Rabbit [0–1]
- Venison [0–1]

Poultry

Lower in saturated fat than many cuts of red meat, poultry is popular and easy to prepare. Much of the fat in poultry is in the skin, so you need to remove it or buy skinless, boneless chicken or turkey. You can cook poultry with skin on and remove it before eating.

- ✔ Chicken, dark meat [3 grams of fat per ounce]
- ✔ Chicken, white meat [0–1]
- ✔ Cornish hen [0–1]
- ✔ Duck, domestic [3]
- ✔ Goose, domestic [3]
- ✔ Pheasant (no skin) [0–1]
- ✔ Turkey, dark meat [3]
- ✔ Turkey, white meat [0–1]

Cholesterol in foods is not the same as cholesterol in your blood. High levels of blood cholesterol can lead to heart disease. The saturated fat in your diet leads to high blood cholesterol more than the cholesterol in foods does.

Eggs

Previously, three eggs a week was the maximum allotted amount because egg yolks were believed to contain as much as 274 mg of cholesterol, practically filling up the daily allotment of 300 mg in one gulp. Today, an egg is known to have around 214 to 220 mg of cholesterol, allowing room in the diet for one egg a day — provided egg-lovers can keep their remaining cholesterol intake below the 300-mg-per-day benchmark.

When eating eggs, keep the rest of your diet low in saturated fat. Eggs have 5 grams of fat per ounce.

If this still seems like too much cholesterol for your diet, you may want to check out some new cholesterol-friendly egg-based products like Eggland's Best and Egg Beaters. Eggland's Best are eggs from hens that are deliberately fed a diet that lowers the eggs' cholesterol significantly, to around 180 mg per egg. Egg Beaters are made primarily from seasoned egg whites (no yolks), making them a handy choice.

The cholesterol is all in the yolk; there is none in the white. If you have the time (and don't want to spend the extra cash for the premade products), you can make your own cholesterol-free egg products. Use two egg whites and 1 teaspoon oil in place of a whole egg in a recipe. If you're making an omelet or frittata, you can probably get away without using the extra oil.

Cheese

Cheese is a nutritious food, but not a low-fat one. Most supermarkets carry reduced-fat cheeses. Try combining cheese with fresh fruit for a healthy snack or dessert.

- Cheddar, reduced-fat [5 grams of fat per ounce]
- Colby, reduced-fat [5]
- Cottage cheese, low-fat [0–1]
- Cottage cheese, regular [3]
- Feta [5]
- Mozzarella [5]
- Parmesan [3]
- Ricotta [5]

Note: Regular cheddar and Colby cheese have 10 grams of fat per ounce! Make sure to choose the reduced-fat variety.

Seafood

Seafood is a terrific source of protein, low in calories and low in fat. Whether you choose fish or shellfish, you're bound to get a dose of concentrated protein, all wrapped up in a light and delicate package.

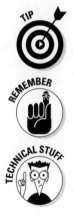

If you're not familiar with including fish in your diet, start with canned tuna and salmon. Then try broiled orange roughy, flounder, tilapia, or grilled salmon. Start ordering grilled, broiled, or baked fish and seafood in restaurants to become familiar with non-fried choices.

Current guidelines from the American Heart Association recommend two seafood-based meals a week for all Americans. Fish is a heart-healthy food because it is high in omega-3 fatty acids.

Omega-3 fatty acids are good fats that make your blood less likely to form clots that can cause a heart attack. Experts recommend that healthy people eat omega-3 fatty acids from fish and plant sources to protect their hearts. The fatty acids also protect against irregular heartbeat that causes sudden cardiac death. Check out Chapter 8 for more about omega-3s and other fatty acids.

Healthy adults should eat two servings a week of fish such as mackerel, lake trout, herring, sardines, albacore tuna, and salmon.

Fish

Fresh fish contains less saturated fat than red meat. Try to eat fish two to three times a week. Most markets have significantly expanded their seafood offerings. Check with your local fishmonger for his recommendations.

- Catfish [3 grams of fat per ounce]
- Cod, fresh or frozen [0–1]
- Flounder [0–1]
- Grouper [0–1]
- Haddock [0–1]
- Halibut [0–1]
- Herring, uncreamed or smoked [3]
- Mahimahi [0–1]
- Mackerel [3]
- Pompano [3]
- Orange roughy [0–1]
- Salmon, fresh or canned [3]
- Sardines, canned [3]
- Scrod [0–1]
- Snapper [0–1]
- Sole [0–1]
- Swordfish [3]
- Trout [0–1]
- Tuna, ahi [0–1]
- Tuna, albacore [0–1]
- Tuna, canned in oil [3]
- Tuna, canned in water [0–1]
- Tuna, yellowfin [0–1]

Shellfish and mollusks

Most shellfish, if not fried, are very low in fat. Shrimp is higher in cholesterol than most other seafood but low in fat.

 ✔ Clams [0–1 grams of fat per ounce]

 ✔ Crab [0–1]

 ✔ Crawfish [0–1]

 ✔ Lobster [0–1]

 ✔ Mussels [0–1]

 ✔ Oysters, raw [0–1]

 ✔ Scallops [0–1]

 ✔ Shrimp [0–1]

Making Meals from Whole-Food Choices

Let Green Light foods be the focus of your meals. Each meal should have a lean meat, fish, or poultry, at least one serving of the free veggies, and at least one serving of the free fruits. ***Remember:*** You aren't held to a specific amount. You could eat grilled chicken, a large leafy green salad, green beans, and a bowl of cantaloupe, and you're still in the Green Light section! Another meal selection could be baked cod, a mixed fresh fruit cup, steamed broccoli and carrots, and fresh spinach and orange salad.

Use snacks for appetite control. Amazingly, many people who battle their weight don't eat often enough! That's right, eat more frequently to lose weight, but choose Green Light foods. I like to call this preventive eating. In other words, you eat in order not to eat. Strategically plan snacks in your day. Raw fruits and veggies make great snacks and satisfy your appetite on their own. However, I've found that the protein foods taste better with a fruit or veggie partner. Here are some examples:

 ✔ String cheese and seedless grapes

 ✔ Chicken salad with light mayonnaise and Granny Smith apples

 ✔ Lettuce-wrapped Chihuahua cheese and salsa

 ✔ Boiled shrimp and zingy tomato cocktail sauce

 ✔ Prosciutto and melon

Sounds really simple, huh? To get you started, use these easy recipes as examples of ways to incorporate the Green Light foods listed in this chapter into a varied, delicious diet. Did I mention these are free foods? That means you can eat them any time you feel like it!

☺ Marilyn's Orange-Pineapple Delight

Here is a recipe for a dish that is a free food on the Whole Foods Eating Plan. You can eat this any time you want and whenever you want. It's a real lifesaver for some people when it comes to satisfying hunger. Often, a small cupful is enough to take the edge off your appetite, giving you more control at mealtime.

Preparation time: *10 minutes*

Cooking time: *None*

Yield: *8 servings*

24-ounce container cottage cheese	*14.5-ounce can pineapple tidbits in pineapple juice, drained well*
1 large package of sugar-free orange gelatin	*½ cup Cool Whip*
11-ounce can mandarin oranges, drained well	

1 Mix the gelatin powder with the cottage cheese until dissolved.

2 Stir in the drained fruits.

3 Add just enough Cool Whip to smooth out the texture. Store in the refrigerator for up to one week.

Vary It! *Make up your own combination of cottage cheese, sugar-free gelatin, and fruit.*

Per serving: *Calories 139 (From Fat 42); Fat 5g (Saturated 3g); Cholesterol 13mg; Sodium 411mg; Carbohydrate 11g (Dietary Fiber 1g); Protein 12g.*

☺ Vegetable Salad

Here is a suggestion for putting together a big salad from the free-vegetable list.

Preparation time: *10 minutes*

Cooking time: *None*

Yield: *5 servings*

5 cups Romaine lettuce, torn in pieces	*2¼-ounce can sliced black olives*	*4 ounces sliced mushrooms*
1 pint cherry tomatoes, sweet grape size, cut in half	*14-ounce can artichoke hearts, drained well, cut in quarters*	*1 small bell pepper, chopped*
		¼ cup low-fat Italian dressing
		4 ounces feta cheese crumbles

1 Toss together all the ingredients except for the feta cheese.

2 Sprinkle with the cheese.

Vary It! *Try different combinations of veggies and cheeses. Or add 1 cup cooked, diced, skinless chicken meat.*

Per serving: Calories 149 (From Fat 70); Fat 8g (Saturated 4g); Cholesterol 20mg; Sodium 755mg; Carbohydrate 14g (Dietary Fiber 5g); Protein 8g.

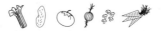

Hearty Vegetable Soup

This hearty soup is great on a cold day. Very filling!

Preparation time: *15 minutes*

Cooking time: *40 minutes*

Yield: *Approximately nine 1½-cup servings*

16-ounce can tomato juice	6 medium carrots, sliced	3 tablespoons Worcestershire sauce
14.5-ounce can fat-free chicken broth	2 cups frozen sliced okra	2 teaspoons Mrs. Dash Table Blend
Two 28-ounce cans diced tomatoes, not drained	1 medium onion, cut in chunks	
	2 cups frozen sliced green beans	

1 Mix the juice, broth, and canned tomatoes in a 3-quart saucepan.

2 Simmer carrots and onions for 10 minutes before adding the frozen and chopped vegetables.

3 Stir in the seasonings.

4 Cook over medium-high heat for 10 minutes. Reduce the heat and simmer for 30 minutes until vegetables are tender.

5 Store in refrigerator for up to one week or freeze to enjoy any time.

Vary It! *To make a hearty meal, add leftover chicken. Try other vegetable combinations like tomatoes, okra, and squash; or cabbage, bell pepper, and mushroom. Anything on the Green Light list is fair game.*

Per serving: Calories 95 (From Fat 0); Fat 0g (Saturated 0g); Cholesterol 0mg; Sodium 580mg; Carbohydrate 22g (Dietary Fiber 6g); Protein 4g.

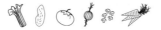

If you like a savory cottage cheese treat, try the Zesty Cottage Cheese recipe in Chapter 11.

Soup tends to taste much better the second or third day, giving flavors time to fully develop. Most soups can be frozen in airtight containers for up to three months. For quick serving, freeze soup in serving-size portions.

Letting Green-Light Foods Satisfy Your Appetite

The trick to eating well is knowing when you've had enough but not too much. You probably recognize that stuffed feeling, and you certainly know when you're still hungry. You also know that both of these states are uncomfortable. The trick is recognizing that just-right state and the feeling of satisfaction that goes with it.

To get a better sense of when you've had enough to eat, but not too much, follow these suggestions:

- **Slow it down.** Your stomach needs 15 minutes to tell your brain that you're full. Eat slowly and let your brain catch up!

- **Forget counting calories.** Focus on feeling satisfied with proper foods instead of targeting a specific calorie value. If you don't feel full, eat more fruits, non-starchy vegetables, or lean protein foods rather than sweets and junk foods.

- **Prepare yourself mentally for making changes in your diet, then set a start date.**

- **Eat regular meals — three meals, three to four hours apart, with three food groups at each meal.**

- **Plan snacks of Green Light foods.**

- **Divide your plate into quarters and fill three quarters with Green Light foods.**

- **Drink six to eight 8-ounce glasses of water per day.**

- **Follow this plan 90 percent of the time, and treat yourself to a favorite food 10 percent of the time.**

The health benefits of eating more fruits and vegetables

You can reduce your risk of coronary heart disease, stroke, and obesity by increasing your consumption of vegetables and fruit. In addition, some scientific studies have demonstrated that greater fruit and vegetable consumption is consistent with a reduced risk of some types of cancers, including cancer of the stomach, esophagus, and lungs. The types of vegetables that most often appear to be protective against cancer are raw vegetables, followed by *allium* vegetables (onions, garlic, scallions, leeks, chives), carrots, green vegetables, *cruciferous* vegetables (broccoli, cauliflower, Brussels sprouts, cabbage), and tomatoes.

Chapter 6

Navigating Your Way through the Starchy Carbs

*P*oor misunderstood carbohydrate. First it was good, and then it was bad. Will these nutrition people make up their minds? I don't blame you if you're frustrated and confused when it comes to carbs. Nutrition science can actually be pretty complex. And to add insult to injury, when nutrition messages are simplified, very important facts often get left out. So, in this chapter I skip the nutrition talk and fast-forward to food. (If you want more details about the science of carbohydrates, check out Chapter 3.)

Of all the many functions of carbohydrate foods, in this chapter I want you to keep one main function in mind: Carbohydrate is fuel. You've probably heard carbs described as a quick-energy food. A lot of people think what that means is, "If I eat carbs, I'll feel more energetic." For most people, that's not exactly true. Marathon runners often eat a lot of pasta before a big race. Why? Because they need a quick energy source to fuel their muscles for their long run ahead. If you're going to sit or stand on the sidelines to cheer them on, do you need a lot of pasta? No. And if you aren't going to burn the fuel, then you'll store the fuel. And guess how that fuel is stored? You got it — as the dreaded body fat.

Any person who is overweight or obese needs to eat less *refined* carbohydrate. Refined carbohydrates are carbs that have been processed to the point of oblivion — well, at least to the point where their nutritive value is diminished and their glycemic index is usually high. Only lean and active people can tolerate a lot of carbohydrate. After you lose weight, if you want to eat more carbs, then you must become more active.

If you sit around all day, you don't need many carbs. If you run around all day, then you can eat more of them.

In this chapter, I show you how to lower the carbohydrate in your diet from refined and starchy food sources to allow for weight loss without sacrificing good nutrition.

Yellow Light: Putting Starchy Carbs on Cruise Control

In the Whole Foods Eating Plan, certain fruits and vegetables are classified as Green Light, meaning "Go, go, go, and eat all you want." These foods are listed in detail in Chapter 5. There *is* carbohydrate in these foods, but it is not counted in the Whole Foods Eating Plan, because it's usually low on the glycemic load index and is very healthy for you. Carbohydrate that comes from starchy food sources is called Yellow Light, meaning "Exercise caution." Be careful not to eat too much of these foods, because you can only have five choices a day. Occasionally, you can substitute a refined or sweet carb for one or two of your starchy carbs.

Controlling your intake of the starchy carbs outlined in this section is a key component of the Whole Foods Eating Plan. This is the feature of the diet that will allow for weight loss and will lower your triglycerides, blood sugar, and blood pressure if they're elevated. You may have five carbohydrate choices per day. A carbohydrate choice is a serving that supplies 15 grams of total carbohydrate — for example, 3 cups of low-fat microwave popcorn or ½ cup of beans. Try to choose the healthiest foods in this category (for example, whole-grain breads and cereals or dried beans and peas).

Because you live in the real world and not just in the pages of this book, the plan is designed to also let you have an occasional sweet treat or snack food. Don't fall into the trap of saying, "I won't eat any of the Yellow Light foods. I can just eat the Green Light foods and lose weight faster." Doing so will put you at risk of insufficient carbohydrate for your needs. Plus, you'll be eliminating some very important healthy foods from your diet.

The goal is to eat well *and* lose weight. Always eat at least three servings of carbs, but no more that five servings from this group per day. Check out the next section for information on how much constitutes a serving.

Controlling Portion Sizes

The key to enjoying carbohydrates while maintaining a low-carb lifestyle is portion control. The Yellow Light foods are not free foods like the delicious cornucopia detailed in Chapter 5. They're categorized as Yellow Light because you need to exercise caution and keep them under control. Exceeding the serving size of a lot of the foods in this category is easy to do.

Breads

Bread is an important part of any healthy diet, even a low-carb one. Over the years, many people have increased their intake of bread because it is low in fat, despite being fairly high in carbs. But the important thing to consider when choosing bread is the type of grain used to make it. Refined-grain breads, like everyday white bread, are soft, smooth-textured, and very tasty. However, refining the grain eliminates a lot of nutrients and increases the glycemic load of the bread, meaning your body converts these carbs to glucose very quickly; thus, you aren't satisfied for long and get hungrier quicker. Whole-grain breads are more nutritious and lower on the glycemic index chart; they affect your blood sugar more slowly and leave you feeling full longer.

Choose whole-grain rolls, muffins, and bread products to stay fuller longer. For more on glycemic index and glycemic load, see Chapter 3 and Appendix B. For more information on the benefits of whole grains and fiber in your diet, take a look at "Choosing the Best, Leaving the Rest," later in this chapter.

Each serving of the following bread items equals approximately 15 grams of total carbohydrate (or one serving).

Food	*Amount to Equal One Serving*
Bagel, small	1
Bread, reduced-calorie (40 calories/slice)	2 slices
Bread, white, whole-wheat, pumpernickel, rye	1 slice
Breadsticks, crisp, 4 inches long by ½ inch thick	2
English muffin	½
Hot dog or hamburger bun	½
Pita, 6 inches across	½

Food	Amount to Equal One Serving
Raisin bread, unfrosted	1 slice
Roll, plain, small	1
Tortilla, corn, 6 inches across	1
Tortilla, flour, 7 to 8 inches across	1
Waffle, 4½ inches square, reduced-fat	1

The more refined a grain is, the fewer the vitamins and minerals and the higher the glycemic load. When you eat these refined foods, they quickly turn to blood sugar. Choose whole, intact grain foods, such as wheat, rye, and barley. They are a major source of cereal fiber and contain numerous phytochemicals that can lower your risk of heart disease, diabetes, and cancer. Eat a minimum of three servings per day.

Cereals, grains, and pasta

The principle of whole grains applies here. Choose whole-grain cereals with no added sugar and whole-wheat pasta. Each serving of these foods equals approximately 15 grams of total carbohydrate (or one serving).

Food	Amount to Equal One Serving
Bran cereals	½ cup
Bulgur	½ cup
Cereals, cooked	½ cup
Cereals, unsweetened, ready-to-eat	¾ cup
Cornmeal, dry	3 tablespoons
Couscous	⅓ cup
Flour, dry	3 tablespoons
Granola, low-fat	¼ cup
Grape-Nuts	¼ cup
Grits	½ cup
Kasha	½ cup
Millet	¼ cup
Muesli	¼ cup
Oats	½ cup
Pasta, macaroni, spaghetti, cooked	½ cup

Food	Amount to Equal One Serving
Puffed cereal	1½ cups
Quinoa	½ cup
Rice, white or brown	⅓ cup
Shredded Wheat	½ cup
Sugar-frosted cereal	½ cup
Wheat germ	3 tablespoons

To bump up your intake of whole-grain foods, look for one of the following ingredients *first* on the food label's ingredient list:

- ✔ Brown rice
- ✔ Oatmeal
- ✔ Whole oats
- ✔ Bulgur
- ✔ Popcorn
- ✔ Whole rye
- ✔ Cracked wheat
- ✔ Whole barley
- ✔ Whole wheat
- ✔ Graham flour
- ✔ Whole cornmeal

Try some of these whole-grain foods:

- ✔ Whole-wheat bread
- ✔ Whole-grain ready-to-eat cereal
- ✔ Low-fat whole-wheat crackers
- ✔ Oatmeal
- ✔ Corn tortillas
- ✔ Whole-wheat pasta
- ✔ Whole barley in soup
- ✔ Tabouli salad

But remember to count each serving of 15 grams of total carbohydrate as one of your five carbohydrate choices.

Quinoa: The super "grain"

Quinoa (KEEN-wah), shown here, isn't exactly a grain, but this wonder food cooks like a grain, tastes like a grain, quacks like a grain. . . . You get the picture. Quinoa is actually a seed that is packed full of protein (including the all-important amino acid, lysine), calcium, and B-complex vitamins, including folic acid.

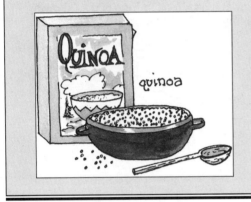

Quinoa is a wonder food with at least as complete a protein as whole milk, and about as many carbs. Relatively new to North America, quinoa sustained the South American Incas, dating back at least 5,000 years. The seed itself closely resembles millet and comes in a variety of colors, ranging from red, orange, and yellow to white and black.

Before arriving at your grocery-store shelves, the seeds are processed to remove their bitter saponin coating. Unlike traditional refining, this process does not diminish the nutritional value of the quinoa; it simply makes it palatable.

You can find quinoa in most health-food stores and many larger grocery stores.

Wheat flour, enriched flour, and degerminated corn meal are not whole grains. Most basic all-purpose or white flour comes from wheat; it's just refined and less healthy. And just because the bread is brown does not mean it's whole-grain. Some food manufacturers just add color to white bread to make it look like whole wheat.

Vegetables and fruit

Starchy vegetables are delicious and you're not alone if you love them. The white Russet potato, a big crowd-pleaser, is particularly high in glycemic load. Enjoy these vegetables, but watch the portion size and count them appropriately as part of your five carbohydrate choices.

Food	Amount to Equal One Serving
Baked beans	⅓ cup
Banana	1 small (6 inches long)
Corn	½ cup
Corn on the cob, medium	1 ear

Food	*Amount to Equal One Serving*
Mixed vegetables with corn, peas, or pasta	1 cup
Peas, green (English peas)	½ cup
Plantain	½ cup
Potato, baked or boiled	1 small
Potato, mashed	½ cup
Squash, winter (acorn, butternut)	1 cup
Yam or sweet potato, plain	½ cup

The banana is one fruit I put on the starch list, because it has a higher starch content than other fruits. Bananas are the number-one fruit sold in the United States, and many people who eat bananas tend to eat a lot of them. So enjoy them occasionally, but be sure to count them as a carbohydrate choice. If you have been told by your doctor to eat bananas for potassium, be aware that you can get just as much potassium from your Green Light fruits and vegetables, such as cantaloupe, orange or grapefruit juice, honeydew, watermelon, raisins, broccoli, spinach, summer squash, and tomatoes.

Dried beans, peas, and lentils

Dried beans and peas contain a fair amount of protein and are often counted as a meat substitute. They're low in glycemic load and can contain as many as 8 grams of dietary fiber per serving.

Here's a list of the portion size of these foods that counts as a carbohydrate choice.

Food	*Amount to Equal One Serving*
Beans and peas (garbanzo, pinto, kidney, white, split, black-eyed)	½ cup
Edamame (green soybeans)	½ cup
Lentils	½ cup
Lima beans	⅔ cup
Miso	3 tablespoons
Peanuts	3 ounces
Tofu, extra-firm	1 cup
Tofu, silken	1 cup

Miso is a soybean paste that is a key ingredient in Japanese cuisine. Use it to quickly add the health benefits of soy to your meals, but watch how much you use if you're watching your blood pressure. This condiment is full of sodium.

Speaking of soy, don't be afraid to try edamame (ed-ah-MAH-may) or green soybeans. You can find these protein-packed pods in the produce department or in the freezer section of most grocery stores. Boiled in lightly salted water, they can satisfy a salty craving without adding much fat or sodium. A half cup has around 15 grams of dietary fiber, 70 mg of calcium, 10 grams of carbs, and 11 grams of protein. Munch away!

If you don't eat animal products, but you want to follow a low-carb diet, use this group of Yellow Light foods as your Green Light proteins. If there is no meat, fish, or poultry at a meal, then the legumes and soy products count as protein, not starch. However, if there is an animal meat at the meal, you have to count these products as starch.

Leery to love legumes?

Maybe the word itself is a little intimidating. Legumes (LEH-gooms) is a fancy word to describe the food family that includes black beans, black-eyed peas, garbanzo beans, Great Northern beans, kidney beans, lentils, navy beans, peanuts, pinto beans, soybeans, and practically any other kind of bean you can think of.

Once scorned as "the poor man's meat," legumes are a nutritional powerhouse. They are an inexpensive, health-promoting, land-sparing, nutritious food. They're full of fiber and protein, and some even contain decent amounts of calcium and very little fat. All legumes add essential vitamins and minerals to your diet.

Because they're relatively inexpensive, many countries and cultures have a long tradition of using them as the staple of their diet. In China and Japan, much of their cooking is related to soybean products, including sprouts, bean curd (tofu), and, of course, soy sauce. In India, lentils, beans, and chickpeas are the number-one protein source in everything from fritters to saucy curries. And what would Latin American cuisine be without black beans and pinto beans? Americans love their peanut butter, baked beans, Texas-style chili with beans, bean sprouts, garbanzo beans, and so on. What French farmhouse is complete without its homemade cassoulet? You get the picture.

Legumes are versatile and easy to prepare. You can find them dried, fresh, canned, or frozen. The canned variety are great for quick meals, but with a pressure cooker, you can have freshly cooked beans in minutes, compared to hours when cooked in the traditional method. Get a variety and find your favorites. Your stomach and intestines will thank you.

Some people do experience gas after eating legumes. Here are a couple of tips to alleviate the problem:

✔ Soak dried legumes overnight, then drain and rinse them before preparing them. This process seems to remove some of the gas-giving components. If using canned beans, just drain and rinse them.

✔ Use a commercially available food enzyme, like Beano. This enzyme helps your body break down the carbohydrate in the legumes so the bacteria in your intestines don't get the chance to break it down and create gas in the process.

Oh, soy good!

You've probably heard a little something about soy. Whether it's soy supplements for menopausal and premenopausal women, or good press about the Asian diet, soy is making more news than ever these days.

Soy foods are packed full of great things including protein, carbs, calcium, vitamins, omega-3 fatty acids, and fiber. You name it, it's probably in there. The protein in soy is complete, meaning it has all eight essential amino acids.

Soy is packed full of antioxidants and isoflavones, which are powerful health-promoting compounds. Soy is believed to help reduce the risk of cardiovascular disease, by helping to lower LDL ("bad") cholesterol, and some kinds of cancer, including breast, prostate, and uterine cancer.

Soy estrogens are helping to alleviate menopausal symptoms for many women.

Preliminary research indicates that soy foods are particularly good for diabetics at risk or experiencing symptoms of kidney disease.

If you haven't taken the plunge, try fitting soy products into your diet. Tofu may not sound appealing to you, but the best thing about it (besides the obvious nutrition) is that it takes on the flavor of whatever your cook it in or with. It's great in soups and sauce. Crumble a little in spaghetti sauce or chili.

Or you may prefer to try a type of soy that's completely different like edamame, miso, soy nuts, or soy milk. So rather than replace meat with tofu, just add soy products to your diet.

Currently, there is no official Recommended Daily Allowance (RDA) for soy protein, but many food producers are calling out soy protein grams separately on their food labels.

Crackers and snacks

This is a category of food that has gotten completely out of hand in the American diet. Most of these foods are made from refined flour and are low in vitamins and minerals. Think about how frequently you choose these foods and try to substitute fresh fruit and veggies for your snack. When you do choose these foods, keep in mind that one serving equals approximately 15 grams of total carbohydrate.

Food	*Amount to Equal One Serving*
Animal crackers	8
Graham crackers, 2½-inch square	3
Matzoh	¾ ounce
Melba toast	4 slices
Oyster crackers	24
Popcorn (popped, no fat added or low-fat microwave)	3 cups (½ bag)

Food	Amount to Equal One Serving
Pretzels	¾ ounce
Rice cakes, 4 inches across	2
Saltine-type crackers	6
Snack chips (tortilla, potato)	15 to 20 (1 ounce)
Soy nuts	1½ ounce
Vanilla wafers	5
Whole-wheat crackers, no fat added	2 to 5 (¾ ounce)

To keep from overeating snack foods, take out the portion you need and then put the bag or box away. That way, you won't reach into a large bag of snacks and continue eating until the bag is empty. Try to include raw fruit, veggies, or low-fat cheese with your snack.

Check out soy nuts if you haven't tried them. You get one and a half to two times the quantity compared to other snacks, plus you add calcium, protein, soy, and dietary fiber wrapped up in a snack-food package. Look for these in the snack-food aisle in many flavors — chile-lime, salt, teriyaki, and even barbecue.

Choosing the Best, Leaving the Rest

A good rule of the thumb for making your carbohydrate selection each day is to stick to low-glycemic-load foods as often as possible. Choose whole grains for at least three of your carb choices and legumes for the other two for the healthiest diet. These foods will satisfy you longer, so you'll need to refuel less often. Occasionally, you can select more refined foods. These foods will satisfy the occasional craving but typically have less fiber, vitamins, minerals, and overall nutrition. And always remember to count both with the appropriate number of carbohydrate choices.

Low-glycemic-load carbs

Foods with a low glycemic load affect your blood sugar slowly. Here are some examples of low-glycemic-load carbs and their serving sizes:

- ½ cup of beans or peas (garbanzo, pinto, kidney, white, split, black-eyed)
- ⅔ cup of lima beans
- 1 slice of high-fiber bread (rye, whole-wheat, multigrain)
- ¾ ounce (2 to 5) whole-wheat crackers
- 3 cups of low-fat microwave popcorn

Whole-grain foods fall into the lower-glycemic-load category because they slow the digestion of starches into the bloodstream. These foods also have many other nutritional benefits, including the following:

- They improve the health of the gastrointestinal tract by improving regularity.

- They lower the risk of mouth, stomach, colon, gallbladder, and ovarian cancer.

- They reduce LDL ("bad") cholesterol, while maintaining HDL ("good") cholesterol.

- They may reduce some kinds of heart disease.

- They contain valuable *phytochemicals* (naturally occurring plant-based chemicals that help fight disease).

- They contain essential vitamins and minerals.

High-glycemic-load carbs

High-glycemic-load carbs quickly affect your blood sugar and may leave you hungrier more quickly than their low-glycemic-load counterparts. Starchy veggies with a high glycemic load like potatoes can be part of your diet and add to your daily fiber intake as long as you eat them in moderation. Stick to the portions outlined earlier in this chapter to ensure you're staying within your daily allotment of carbohydrate choices.

Whenever possible, eat your starchy vegetables, like potatoes, with the skin intact. You're sure to get the most nutrients and an extra dose of dietary fiber. Better nutrition and a full tummy — what more could you ask for? Don't go crazy and start eating banana peels and spaghetti squash hulls, because that's just, well, silly — but eating a russet potato skin now and then won't hurt you.

Here are some examples of carbohydrate choices with a higher glycemic load:

- 1 slice white bread

- ½ cup of macaroni, spaghetti, or rice

- ½ cup of potatoes

- ¾ cup of unsweetened, ready-to-eat cereal

- 6 saltine crackers

- 5 vanilla wafers

For more on the glycemic load and glycemic index of foods, check out Appendix B.

Putting the Brakes on Refined Carbs

Refined carbs are foods that are highly processed and pre-packaged, like chips, cookies, cakes, candy, crackers, and bread. They may even have enticing packaging, claiming to be fat-free or cholesterol-free. But be very discriminating and read your nutrition labels so you know exactly what you're eating. (See Chapter 9 for more information on reading food labels the low-carb way.) You'll eat *some* refined carbs. You just don't want to eat them too frequently or in too great a quantity.

Refined carbohydrates have a low nutrient density, meaning their nutrient value is low compared to the number of calories they pack. Many of these foods have become popular because they're low in fat. People see them as free foods because of their low fat grams, a big mistake.

When you do choose these foods, reduce your intake of the other carbohydrate foods to maintain balance and control in your eating. If you've spent your carbs for the day, remember you can still eat those Green Light foods in Chapter 5 — fruits, veggies, and lean proteins.

Trading off your carb choices for an occasional treat

Okay, so how do you handle a potato-chip craving that just can't be cured by microwave low-fat popcorn? Or what happens when the pop machine is out of no-calorie soda? Don't panic, just readjust your carbohydrate choices for the day with a trade-off. One snack-size (1-ounce) bag of potato chips has 16 grams of total carbohydrate, so you can trade one of your five carbohydrate choices for this puny bag.

One 12-ounce can of regular soda has 40 grams of total carbohydrate (and it's 100-percent sugar and 0-percent nutrients). If you choose a can of regular soda, count it as two and a half of your carb choices for the day. It's okay to make that kind of trade occasionally, but when you do, you can only have two and a half carbohydrate choices for the rest of the day — not very many.

Let's say you're at a coworker's birthday party. You're handed a piece of birthday cake and you want to eat it. If it's a normal size serving of birthday cake, just count it as two carb choices and go on about your day. Now, if that unintended birthday cake means you've had your five carb choices by mid-afternoon, then no more carbs for you. *Remember:* On the Whole Foods Eating Plan, you can still eat your Green Light fruits, veggies, and lean proteins.

These trade-offs may sound appealing, and you may be plotting your first trade-off as you read. But you can't underestimate the long-term detriment to your health of making these trade-offs too often. Without the critical fiber and nutrition you need daily, your general health and weight will suffer.

When evaluating the food labels of trade-off foods, here's a chart to help you work out your own trade-offs. (*Remember:* You can subtract the dietary fiber out of the total carb on the food label.) Check out Chapter 9 for more information on counting total carbohydrate.

Total Carbohydrate	*Starch Count*
6 to 10 grams	½ carb
11 to 19 grams	1 carb
20 to 25 grams	1½ carbs
26 to 35 grams	2 carbs

If your item has less than 5 grams of carbs per serving *and* you eat only one serving, don't count the carbs. Just keep in mind that a lot of 5-gram carb portions can add up in a day. So don't go crazy with this.

The Nutrition Facts panel tells you how much *total* carbohydrate is in one serving. This includes the amount attributed to dietary fiber. You may subtract the dietary fiber from the total carbohydrate amount. Then calculate the number of carb choices per serving. For more on deciphering food labels, turn to Chapter 9.

Paying attention to sugar

You can eat sweets and sugar, if you count the carbohydrate they contain. The problem is that sugars and sweets don't have vitamins or minerals, and they do have a lot of calories, even in small servings. My best recommendation is to avoid hidden sugars in food, especially refined, pre-packaged, and processed foods. Make the sugar you eat count. Did you really enjoy that fat-free cookie? Probably not, but it likely contained 12 grams of carbs, which is equivalent to eating an entire *tablespoon* of sugar. You'd probably be more satisfied with ¾ cup of fresh strawberries, which contain the same number of carbs, have way more fiber and nutrients, and are pretty darn filling. And don't forget, strawberries are free to you — whereas the fat-free cookie will cost you one carb choice for the day.

Many foods contain both carbohydrate and fat, including sweets, such as cakes, pies, cookies, candy, ice cream, jelly, chocolate, and snack foods, such as chips and crackers.

Avoiding the urge to exceed your daily allowance

The best way to avoid exceeding the carb allowance is to build your meals around the Green Light foods. Always think of those free fruits and veggies first because the amounts are unlimited. Also track your portion sizes of carb choice foods. Overeating of a particular food is often a habit. It's surprising how satisfying a smaller portion can be, especially if you eat it with a variety of unlimited foods. If nothing seems to abate that sweet craving, then indulge it with a controlled amount. Eat it slowly, savor it, and then get back on track. You can compensate for what you've eaten by dropping a couple of carbs or increasing your exercise that day.

Fitting in Your Daily Dietary Fiber

Fiber is an important contribution from many of the foods in this group. Soluble fiber is helpful in lowering your cholesterol and comes from whole grains like oats, barley, and rye and also from dried beans and peas. Insoluble fiber is helpful in lowering your risk of colon cancer and other cancers of the gastrointestinal tract. Whole grains on the average provide 3 grams of dietary fiber per serving. Specialty cereals designed to provide more fiber (for example, Bran Flakes, All Bran, Fiber One) can provide 8 to 13 grams of dietary fiber per serving. Dried beans and peas can provide up to 8 grams of dietary fiber per serving. If you carefully select foods from this group, you can get the dietary fiber per day that your body needs.

Current dietary fiber guidelines

The latest guidelines from the National Academy of Sciences recommend that women up to the age of 50 include 25 grams and men up to the age of 50 include 38 grams of fiber in their diet every day. Women over age 50 need 21 grams and men over age 50 need 30 grams of dietary fiber per day. Considering that the average person consumes 10 to 12 grams of fiber per day, this is quite an increase. Getting to the recommended level takes careful selection of the five carbohydrate servings. Don't forget to load up on the free fruits and veggies outlined in Chapter 5. They're chock-full of fiber and don't count as any (not one) of your daily carbohydrate choices.

Here are some examples of how to get the most fiber from your five carbohydrate choices:

  ½ cup cooked oatmeal = 3 grams dietary fiber

  1 slice multigrain bread = 2 grams dietary fiber

¾ ounce (5) whole-wheat crackers = 2 grams fiber

3 cups low-fat microwave popcorn = 3 grams fiber

½ cup pinto beans = 8 grams dietary fiber

Total = 5 carb choices and 18 grams of dietary fiber

Add this to the 2 to 4 grams of dietary fiber that you get from each serving of the fruits and vegetables you eat, and you can easily meet the minimum recommendation of 25 grams of fiber for women up to age 50. Men may need a daily serving of the special high-fiber cereals to meet the higher recommendation of 38 grams of fiber for men up to age 50.

To estimate your dietary fiber intake, use the following guide. For more-specific information, check the food label or use a reliable reference.

Food	*Amount*	*Grams of Fiber*
Fruits and vegetables	½ cup cooked; 1 medium piece; or 1 to 2 cups raw	2 to 3
Starchy vegetables	½ cup	3
Legumes	½ cup	6 to 8
Cereals	½ to ¾ cup	2 to 4
Special high-fiber cereals	⅓ to ½ cup	8 to12
Breads and crackers, whole-grain	1 slice or 1 ounce	2 to 3
Nuts and seeds	½ ounce	1 to 2

Located at the Berkeley Nutrition Services Web site (www.nutritionquest. com) is a free Fruit/Veg/Fiber dietary screener that gives you a good estimate of the amount of fiber in your diet. It is quick and easy to use. If you aren't sure where you stand, visit the site to find out more.

If you can't get excited about ½ cup of All-Bran or Fiber One, mix them with ½ to ¾ cup Cheerios or Wheaties for two carb servings and 15 grams of fiber. Add 1 cup fresh strawberries and 1 cup skim milk. You still have only used 2 carb choices and your fiber intake is 19 grams for one meal.

If your usual diet is the typical 10 to 12 grams of dietary fiber, don't go to 25 to 38 grams of fiber overnight. Your intestinal tract will rebel and you'll experience gas, bloating, and discomfort. Instead, start gradually, adding about 3 extra grams of fiber per day, giving your system time to adjust. Also, when increasing fiber intake, remember to drink 6 to 8 glasses of fluid per day.

Putting It on the Menu: The Daily Plan

As a rule, the best way to spend your five carb choices is to pick three of them from the whole-grains family (like whole-wheat crackers or whole-grain bread) and two of them from the legume group (like black beans or lentils) for the fiber. On occasion, you can definitely work in potatoes and bananas and so on. But really work on improving your intake of whole grains and legumes. You'll see results in both weight loss and general good health.

Here's a sample day to get you started. For more on menu planning see Chapter 10.

Breakfast:

½ cup Fiber One cereal (12 grams fiber) sprinkled with toasted almonds (1 gram fiber)

1 cup ½-percent milk

Fresh strawberries (4 grams fiber per cup) sweetened with Splenda

Carbohydrate choices: 1

Lunch:

Turkey sandwich:

2 slices whole-wheat bread (4 grams fiber)

Deli-style turkey breast

1 tablespoon reduced-fat mayonnaise

Mustard

Lettuce

Sliced tomatoes

½ sliced avocado

Orange sections (4 grams fiber per cup)

Iced tea, Splenda optional

Carbohydrate choices: 2

Dinner:

Grilled salmon

Grilled mushrooms, bell peppers, and onions (2 grams fiber)

½ cup wild rice (2 grams fiber)

½ cup pinto bean salad (6 grams fiber)

Watermelon chunks (1 gram fiber per cup)

Carbohydrate choices: 2

Snack:

6 ounces low-fat fruit-flavored yogurt

Total carbohydrate choices for the day: 5

Total fiber: 36 grams (24 grams from the carb choices, 12 from the fruits, veggies, and nuts)

Still hungry? Eat more strawberries, orange sections, or watermelon; veggies; or a little extra turkey meat or salmon. Or try any of the totally free, Green Light recipes in Chapters 11 and 12, like Eggplant Casserole, Savory Carrots, or Ham and Artichoke Bites.

Chapter 7

Shifting into Dairy Foods

In This Chapter

▶ Knowing what you stand to gain from dairy foods

▶ Recognizing the importance of calcium in your diet

▶ Making sure you're getting enough calcium

T hink only babies and young children need milk? Do you shun dairy foods when you're dieting because you think they're high in fat? If you answered yes to either question, you're not alone — and you're also mistaken. The nutrients provided by dairy foods are as important when you're old as when you're young. And exciting new research indicates that calcium provided by dairy foods may help you lose weight!

In this chapter, I fill you in on the importance of dairy foods in your diet, focusing in particular on the benefits of calcium (and the risks you face if you aren't getting enough of it). I also let you know how to get calcium from other non-dairy sources.

Understanding the Benefits of Dairy Foods

Dairy foods such as milk, yogurt, cheese, and ice cream contain carbohydrate in the form of a milk sugar called *lactose*. Lactose is the principal carbohydrate of milk, making up about 5 percent of its weight. Lactose contributes 30 to 50 percent of milk's energy, depending on the milk's fat content. However, milk, yogurt, and other dairy products are low in glycemic load, so you can include them in your lower-carbohydrate meal plan. You are allowed two to three servings per day and you do not count them as a carbohydrate choice on the Whole Foods Eating Plan. Check out Chapter 2 for an overview of the eating plan. (For more information on glycemic load and its role in the foods you eat, turn to Chapter 3 and Appendix B.)

The fact that dairy products are low in glycemic load is a good thing, because eating dairy foods has been demonstrated to reduce *hypertension* (high blood pressure), and the risk of osteoporosis, kidney stones, and colon cancer. The fat in dairy products is mostly saturated fat, which can increase the risk of heart disease, but very-low-fat dairy foods and nonfat dairy foods allow you to have all the benefits without the fat. These dairy foods are also rich sources of vital nutrients that can prevent disease. Exciting new research is connecting the calcium from dairy products with weight loss (see the nearby sidebar, "Calcium's role in weight loss," for more information).

Lactose intolerance

Lactose intolerance occurs when the body doesn't make enough of an enzyme called *lactase*. Lactase breaks down lactose (milk sugar) found in dairy foods. When people don't have enough lactase, they may have a problem digesting dairy products. Soon after eating or drinking dairy products, they may experience gas, bloating, stomach cramps, and/or diarrhea. If you're lactose intolerant, you can control the symptoms through simple changes in your diet.

If you avoid dairy products, you may not be getting enough calcium and vitamin D. Both are necessary for healthy bones and the prevention of osteoporosis, a disease that weakens bones and causes them to break easily. To make sure you're getting enough calcium, try these tips:

✔ **Don't give up on dairy entirely.** People who have trouble digesting lactose can often tolerate milk with meals. Start with small ½-cup servings and gradually increase the size of servings. Always drink milk with food; dairy products may be better digested if eaten with other foods, so eat dairy foods with a meal. Try eating smaller quantities of dairy more often; you may be able to tolerate small

amounts of dairy better than a large amount all at once. Eat cheese, which is lower in lactose; aged hard cheeses like Colby, cheddar, Swiss, and parmesan have less lactose than softer cheeses. (Try low-fat versions of these cheeses.) Try yogurt and milk with active cultures, which produce lactase and are often easier to tolerate.

✔ **Look for lactose-free or lactose-reduced dairy foods in your supermarket.**

✔ **Try adding lactase to your food.** Lactase comes in a liquid form, chewable tablets, and capsules. You can buy lactase at your pharmacy without a prescription.

✔ **Eat soy products, which are great sources of calcium.** Try calcium-fortified soy milk, tofu, soy yogurt, and soy nuts.

✔ **Eat lots of dark green leafy vegetables like broccoli, collard greens, kale, turnip greens, mustard greens, and bok choy, all of which are a good source of calcium.**

✔ **Try calcium-fortified juices and calcium-fortified cereals.**

TECHNICAL STUFF

Calcium's role in weight loss

The mineral calcium is a must for healthy bones, but recent studies also show you could lose more weight by adding more calcium to your weight-loss plan. As dietary calcium intake increases, calcium levels within fat cells decrease. In turn, lower calcium levels within cells impact the metabolism of fat, in favor of weight loss. Fat synthesis decreases and fat breakdown increases. This shift in fat metabolism may result in less fat storage and a reduction in body weight.

In other words, getting enough calcium from dairy foods seems to trigger the body to burn more fat and make it harder for new fat cells to form. Of course, calcium can't work alone, but it is effective when combined with the rest of your weight-loss eating plan.

How much calcium do you need in order to lose weight? One major study showed weight loss enhancement with 1,200 mg of calcium provided by dairy foods in the daily diet. Researchers continue to study the role of calcium in a reduced-calorie diet. Meanwhile, getting at least the recommended 1,000 mg of calcium per day from low-fat dairy products, calcium-fortified foods and beverages, and calcium-containing plant foods is a good idea.

Got milk? Got nutrients

Dairy foods are excellent sources of calcium, phosphorous, riboflavin, protein, magnesium, vitamin A, vitamin B_6, and vitamin B_{12}. If fortified (and most milk *is* fortified), milk provides appreciable amounts of vitamin D as well.

So what does this mean for your body? Take a look at just some of the benefits you stand to gain from the nutrients found in dairy products:

- **Phosphorus:** This is an important mineral in bones and teeth and a part of every cell in the body.

- **Riboflavin:** This vitamin supports normal vision and healthy skin. It's important to the production of energy in your body.

- **Protein:** This nutrient builds and repairs body tissues.

- **Magnesium:** This mineral is important in building healthy bones and teeth. It's also important in muscle contractions and nerve impulses.

- **Vitamin A:** This is an important vitamin in maintaining healthy eyes and skin. It is also important in bone and tooth growth.

- **Vitamin B_6:** This vitamin helps make red blood cells and helps build proteins in your body.

✔ **Vitamin B₁₂:** This vitamin prevents anemia and helps maintain healthy nerve cells.

✔ **Vitamin D:** This vitamin helps maintain calcium and phosphorus for healthy bones.

If you were paying attention, you may have noticed calcium missing from that list. That's because the following section is devoted to the benefits of calcium (and what happens to your body if you don't get enough of it).

Calcium: It's everywhere!

Calcium is found in great abundance in the human body, and 99 percent of it is found in the bones and teeth. (That's why, when kids are growing, they need calcium to build strong bones and teeth.) But where is that remaining 1 percent of calcium found? In the blood. Calcium plays important roles in nerve conduction, muscle contraction, and blood clotting.

Knowing how much calcium you need

If calcium levels in the blood drop below normal, your body will pull calcium from your bones and put it into the blood in order to maintain the blood calcium levels it needs. If your blood borrows too much calcium from your bones, you're at risk for lots of conditions related to calcium deficiency, including osteoporosis. Consuming enough calcium throughout your lifetime, whether you're a man or a woman, is important in order to maintain adequate blood and bone calcium levels.

Check out Table 7-1 to see how much calcium and vitamin D you need every day (see the nearby sidebar, "Vitamin D and calcium: Their critical connection," for more information). These guidelines are the same for both men and women.

Table 7-1	The Amount of Calcium and Vitamin D You Need	
Age	*Calcium*	*Vitamin D*
1 to 3 years	500 mg	200 IU
4 to 8 years	800 mg	200 IU
9 to 18 years	1,300 mg	200 IU
19 to 50 years	1,000 mg	200 IU
51 to 70 years	1,200 mg	400 IU

Age	Calcium	Vitamin D
71 years and older	1,200 mg	600 IU
Pregnant or lactating women under 19 years old	1,300 mg	200 IU
Pregnant or lactating women 19 and older	1,000 mg	200 IU

Source: National Academy of Sciences (NAS), 1997

The National Institute of Health Consensus Conference and the National Osteoporosis Foundation recommend a higher calcium intake of 1,500 mg per day for postmenopausal women not taking estrogen and men and women 65 years or older. Talk to your doctor or registered dietitian about the amount of calcium that's right for you.

Although calcium offers many benefits, the old adage "If some is good, more is better" most definitely does not apply. If you take more than 2,500 mg of calcium per day, you may experience adverse side effects. High calcium intakes can lead to constipation and an increased chance of developing calcium kidney stones; it may also inhibit your absorption of iron and zinc, both of which are vital nutrients your body needs. Calcium supplements are better absorbed in divided doses. So, don't take 1200 mg all at one time. Divide it into 600 mg in the morning and 600 mg at night.

If you're a nursing mother whose doctor or lactation consultant has recommended that you cut back on your intake of dairy products because they're upsetting your baby's stomach, make sure you still get at least your minimum calcium requirement from non-dairy sources and supplements. Sufficient calcium in your diet is essential in order to provide proper nutrition for you and your baby. For tips on non-dairy calcium sources, turn to Table 7-3, later in this chapter.

Recognizing what can happen if you don't get enough calcium

Calcium is a principal mineral provided by dairy foods. Everybody needs calcium, but as you age you need even more because your body naturally loses calcium *and* has a much tougher time absorbing it. Talk about a double whammy! Although dairy foods are a rich source of calcium, you can also get calcium from oranges, broccoli, dried beans, soy, spinach, and canned salmon with bones. See Table 7-3 later in this chapter for specifics.

Calcium can play a major role in disease prevention. Three good reasons to count on calcium are the prevention of osteoporosis, high blood pressure, and colon cancer.

TECHNICAL STUFF

Vitamin D and calcium: Their critical connection

Most foods that are fortified with calcium are also fortified with vitamin D. Vitamin D is a critical piece in the calcium-absorption puzzle. It enables your body to use the calcium you're taking in. Additionally, vitamin D helps your body reabsorb calcium in the kidneys rather than allow it to be removed from the body with waste. Vitamin D also helps your body maintain a proper balance of calcium and phosphorous in the bloodstream.

Current guidelines indicate that most people need between 200 and 600 IU (international units) of Vitamin D daily, depending on their age. Vitamin D supplements are usually not necessary because vitamin D is available from fortified milk and foods such as fish and egg yolks.

Vitamin D is also known as "the sunshine vitamin." You only need 15 minutes of sunlight exposure without sunscreen each day to maintain an adequate vitamin D level. The amount of skin exposed to the sun should be the equivalent of your face and arms. Sunscreens with an *SPF* (skin protection factor) of 8 or higher will block vitamin D absorption. Persons living in climates with year round cloudiness blocking the sun's rays will have less vitamin D absorption.

Vitamin D has been shown to produce adverse side effects such as *calcification* (hardening) of soft tissues (blood vessels, heart, lungs, kidneys, tissues around joints) at above 50 mcg or 2,000 IU a day. Take a look at Table 7-1 earlier in this chapter to determine how much vitamin D you need.

To make sure you're getting enough vitamin D in your diet, take a look at some good sources of vitamin D:

Food	Serving Size	Vitamin D
Egg yolk	1 yolk	25 IU
Salmon	3 ounces	425 IU
Fortified milk	1 cup	100 IU
Fortified cereal	½ to 1 cup	40 IU
Sardines	3 ounces	255 IU

Osteoporosis

Osteoporosis means "porous bone." It is a disease characterized by a decrease in bone mineral density and bone calcium content. What does osteoporosis mean in practical terms? It leads to an increased risk of fractures. One out of two women and one out of eight men will develop osteoporosis. A diet high in calcium can help slow bone loss. Preserving bone mass helps reduce your risk of developing this bone-thinning and debilitating disease.

Using calcium supplements

As with any nutrient, food is always your best source of calcium because it is accompanied by additional essential nutrients that benefit your body. If your physician or registered dietitian recommends a calcium supplement, keep in mind that your body will absorb the calcium best if you take it with a meal.

Calcium in foods and in supplements occurs in a compound form. A *compound* is a substance that contains more than one ingredient. Calcium's most likely companions in a compound are carbonate and citrate.

The calcium in a compound is called *elemental calcium*. During digestion, the calcium compound dissolves and the elemental calcium becomes available to be absorbed into the blood. If a tablet contains 500 mg of calcium carbonate, it contains only 200 mg of elemental calcium. This is because only 40 percent of the calcium compound is elemental calcium; the other 60 percent, or 300 mg, is from the carbonate ingredient. Most calcium supplements list the elemental calcium content on the label. The elemental calcium is what counts toward your calcium total for the day.

Calcium carbonate is the most common type of calcium supplement on the market. It's found in products like Tums, Caltrate, and Os-Cal and usually requires extra stomach acid for digestion, so you should take it with a meal. Calcium citrate is another type of calcium supplement, found in products like Citrucal and most calcium-fortified juices. Calcium citrate contains 21 percent elemental calcium. Calcium citrate is the best absorbed supplemental form and does not require the presence of extra stomach acid to dissolve. It is much more expensive than calcium carbonate, so discuss the pros and cons of each type of calcium supplement with your health-care provider.

Those at greater risk of developing osteoporosis include:

✔ People with a low calcium and vitamin D intake (see the preceding section for recommendations on how much calcium and vitamin D you need)

✔ Caucasian or Asian females

✔ Females of any race who are thin and/or small-framed or who weigh less than 127 pounds

✔ People over 65 years of age

✔ People with a family history of osteoporosis

✔ Women who are postmenopausal or who have had a hysterectomy and who are not on estrogen replacement therapy

✔ People with a history of eating disorders

✔ People who regularly follow a low-calorie diet of 1,200 calories or less

✔ Women who are currently having or have had irregular periods or an absence of menstrual periods (lasting more than one year)

✔ People with an inactive lifestyle

✔ People who smoke cigarettes

✔ People who drink more than two alcoholic drinks per day

✔ Men with low testosterone levels

✔ People who regularly use steroid or glucocorticoid medications (such as prednisone or cortisone) for treatment of asthma, arthritis, lupus, or another chronic disease

The more risk factors you have, the greater your risk of developing osteoporosis. Obviously, some risk factors — like your age, your gender, your race, and your family history — you can't do anything about. But you can and should consider the risk factors that are within your control. If you smoke, quit (not just because of osteoporosis, but for your overall health). If you drink heavily, cut back. If you lead an inactive lifestyle, become more active. And obviously, you can increase your intake of dairy products and calcium supplements. Making these kinds of lifestyle changes offers many health benefits, but lowering your risk of osteoporosis is a big one.

High blood pressure

As many as 50 million Americans have high blood pressure (also referred to as *hypertension*). High blood pressure increases your risk of heart disease, stroke, and kidney disease. Calcium, potassium, and magnesium are three nutrients shown to reduce blood pressure. New research shows that increasing your calcium consumption to at least the recommended levels for your age (see "Knowing how much calcium you need," earlier in this chapter) is associated with a small but important reduction in blood pressure. Potassium and magnesium help calcium lower blood pressure. Dairy foods contain ample amounts of all three of these nutrients. Getting all these nutrients in your diet can reduce your systolic blood pressure (the top number in a blood pressure measurement) by 8 to 14 points. Adding exercise will reduce it 4 to 9 points more.

Colon cancer

Colon cancer is the third leading cause of cancer deaths in the United States. A recent study showed that people who consume at least a moderate amount of calcium in their diet (700 to 800 mg per day) significantly reduced their risk of colon cancer by 40 to 50 percent. Boosting your calcium intake, along with consuming a high-fiber diet, may help reduce your risk.

Getting Enough Calcium

The fat in dairy foods contains a high ratio of saturated fat, and high saturated fat intake has consistently been linked to high cholesterol levels and heart disease. Reducing your saturated fat intake as much as possible is a good idea.

TIP

Opt for low-fat or fat-free milk, yogurt, and cheese whenever possible. They contain fewer calories and little to no saturated fat but all the vitamins and minerals that the higher-fat versions contain.

REMEMBER

Children under 2 years of age need quite a bit of fat in their diet for adequate brain and nerve development, so they should drink whole milk instead of the low-fat or fat-free versions.

WHOLE FOODS

Two to three servings per day of fat-free or low-fat dairy foods are allowed on the Whole Foods Eating Plan. However, based on new evidence and a person's individual risk for osteoporosis, three to four servings may be more appropriate for some people. A serving is 1 cup of skim milk, 1 to 1½ ounces of cheese, or 6 to 8 ounces of yogurt.

No matter which number of servings is right for you, make sure your other food choices bring you in line with your minimum calcium requirements for your age.

Here's an example of how to fit your two to three servings in each day and add other foods to hit a 1,200 mg requirement:

- ✓ **Breakfast:** Add 1 cup of skim milk to your whole-grain cereal (302 mg calcium).
- ✓ **Lunch:** Toss a piece of low-fat string cheese into your lunchbox (183 mg calcium). Add a cup of raw broccoli (47 mg calcium).
- ✓ **Afternoon snack:** Enjoy a container of nonfat or low-fat yogurt (400 mg calcium). Add some soy nuts for a quick salty treat (119 mg calcium).
- ✓ **Dinner:** Try some braised kale as a side dish (180 mg calcium).

As you can tell from the preceding list, both dairy and non-dairy foods can be good sources of calcium. Try to include calcium-rich foods from a variety of sources. To get you started, Table 7-2 lists appropriate serving sizes of some common dairy foods and their contribution to your daily calcium tally, and Table 7-3 lists non-dairy calcium-rich options. Many of the non-dairy foods are Green Light foods on the Whole Foods Eating Plan.

Making occasional substitutions

The Whole Foods Eating Plan also allows for occasional substitutions of sugar-free ice cream or frozen yogurt for an occasional treat. These treats should not exceed 90 to 130 calories per serving. Keep in mind that these are calorie-equivalent substitutions and they don't include the same nutrients as a cup of skim milk, so you don't want to be making these substitutions frequently.

Many food manufacturers are capitalizing on the trend of increasing calcium in the diet and have fortified tons of food (literally!) with calcium, including ice cream and water. Although I don't consider these to be great sources of calcium, if you're going to splurge and eat it anyway, you may as well get a little calcium boost. Many of the Healthy Choice no-sugar-added ice creams contain as much as 200 mg of calcium per cup. Always double-check the nutrition label for the full "scoop" before you buy.

Table 7-2	Calcium-Rich Dairy Foods	
Dairy Food	*Serving Size*	*Calcium*
Buttermilk	1 cup	285 mg
Cheese, American	1 ounce	174 mg
Cheese, cheddar	1 ounce	204 mg
Cheese, mozzarella, part-skim	1 ounce	183 mg
Cheese, parmesan	1 tablespoon	69 mg
Cheese, Swiss	1½ ounces	408 mg
Cottage cheese, low-fat	1 cup	155 mg
Frozen yogurt, vanilla	1 cup	103 mg
Ice cream, hard	1 cup	168 mg
Milk, calcium-fortified	1 cup	500 mg
Milk, lactose-free, low-fat	1 cup	300 mg
Milk, skim	1 cup	302 mg
Milk, 2 percent	1 cup	297 mg
Ricotta cheese	½ cup	257 mg
Yogurt, fruited, low-fat	1 cup	314 mg
Yogurt, plain, low-fat	1 cup	400 mg

Table 7-3	Calcium-Rich Non-Dairy Foods	
Food	*Serving Size*	*Calcium*
Protein Foods		
Almonds	⅓ cup	120 mg
Pinto beans	½ cup	40 mg
Salmon (pink), canned, with bones	3 ounces	174 mg
Sardines, with bones	3 ounces	371 mg
Shrimp, canned	3 ounces	50 mg
Soy cheese, calcium-fortified	1 ounce	200 mg
Soy milk, calcium-fortified	1 cup	300 mg
Soy nuts, roasted, salted	½ cup	119 mg
Soy yogurt, calcium-fortified	⅔ cup	500 mg
Soybeans, boiled	1 cup	262 mg
Tempeh	½ cup	77 mg
Tofu, firm, calcium-fortified	½ cup	258 mg
Fruits and Vegetables		
Bok choy	1 cup	160 mg
Broccoli	½ cup	47 mg
Carrots	1 cup	48 mg
Collard greens, cooked	1 cup	358 mg
Kale, cooked	1 cup	180 mg
Mustard greens	1 cup	152 mg
Orange	1 medium	52 mg
Orange juice, calcium-fortified	½ cup	150 mg
Turnip greens	1 cup	250 mg

Calcium contents can vary, especially in calcium-fortified foods. Check the nutrition label. Good sources of calcium are those that provide 20 to 30 percent of the daily value (DV) for calcium.

Chapter 8

Fueling Up with Fats: Good Fats, Bad Fats

Guess what? Fats are back, and some of them are even good for you — so good for you, in fact, that you should eat *more* of them. Eat more fat? Am I crazy? No, despite what my son thinks, I'm not. The concept of eating less fat is so thoroughly ingrained in U.S. culture that anyone encouraging more fat is looked upon with suspicion. For the past 40 years, fat has been treated as public enemy number one. Some Americans got the message and successfully reduced their fat intake from 40 percent of calories to 34 percent of calories, but at the same time, others who reduced their fat intake increased their calorie intake (mainly by eating more carbohydrates). What did that do for our health? As a nation, we're fatter than ever. (For more on this phenomenon, check out Chapter 3.)

In this chapter, I tell you about two different (but very much related) concepts: fat, the nutrient, that functions in your body, and dietary fat that you eat, which may help or hurt your body. I show you how fats that naturally occur in some foods are actually very healthy for you *and* your heart. I introduce you to fats that are absolutely delicious and fun to eat — they not only satisfy your appetite, but also improve your health.

Recognizing How Fat Helps Your Body

Fat has negative connotations for many people, but in the body, fat is an essential nutrient. In fact, fat, in moderate amounts, is *necessary* for your health. In this section, I show you how fat helps your body.

Regulating body processes

All humans need fat in order to maintain healthy skin and regulate choles-terol metabolism. Fat is also necessary for the formation of hormone-like substances called *prostaglandins,* which regulate many body processes such as your body's inflammation response to injury and infection as well as blood vessel contractions and nerve impulses. The fat-soluble vitamins A, D, E, and K, stored in your body fat, play many specific roles in the growth and maintenance of your body.

Providing energy

Fat is a concentrated source of energy for the body by providing 9 calories per gram (compared with 4 calories per gram from either carbohydrates or protein). Fat is an important calorie source especially for infants and young children; 50 percent of the calories in human breast milk come from fat. Some storage of energy in your body in the form of fat is essential to your health.

Storing it up

The body uses whatever fat it needs for energy, and the rest is stored in vari-ous fatty tissues. Some fat is found in blood plasma and other body cells, but the largest amount is stored in the body's fat cells. These fat deposits not only act as storage for energy, but also are important in insulating the body and supporting and cushioning organs.

Understanding the Different Kinds of Fat

Many people assume that dietary fat is directly connected with body fat and heart disease, but that isn't exactly true. Some studies show that women who eat the least amount of fat are the most overweight. As far as heart disease, some fats actually *protect* the heart, while others can certainly be harmful. So, just as not all carbohydrates are created equal, not all fats are created equal. Knowing the differences between the various kinds of fat and identifying where they're found in the foods you eat is key.

Fats are classified in three main categories: saturated, monounsaturated, and polyunsaturated. They differ primarily in the amount of hydrogen they con-tain. The degree of saturation determines whether the fat is a solid or a liquid at room temperature. The basic unit of a fat is called a *fatty acid.* Fats with lots of saturated fatty acids (like butter and lard) are more solid at room temperature; oils (like olive oil and canola oil) contain mostly unsaturated fatty acids and are liquid at room temperature.

The fat in food is often referred to as saturated, monounsaturated, and polyunsaturated, but no dietary fat is 100 percent of any of those categories. Dietary fat is classified by the fatty acid that is present in the greatest quantity. For example, olive oil contains 13 percent saturated fat, 72 percent monounsaturated fat, and 8 percent polyunsaturated fat. Because it contains more monounsaturated fat than anything else, it is classified as a monounsaturated fat.

HDL is "good" cholesterol. It helps keep the arteries clear by picking up fatty fragments and taking them back to the liver where they are degraded. LDL is "bad" cholesterol. This type of cholesterol sticks to your arteries and forms plaque; the result can be reduced blood flow or the formation of a clot that totally blocks blood flow in an artery.

Having trouble remembering which is the "good" and which is the "bad" cholesterol? Try this:

- **HDL cholesterol:** H = *H*ealthy, and you want it *h*igh (the higher the better, but at least above 40 mg/dl)
- **LDL cholesterol:** L = *L*ousy, and you want it *l*ow (the lower the better, but at least below 130 mg/dl) *Note:* If you have diabetes or heart disease, your LDL cholesterol needs to be below 100 mg/dl.

Saturated fats

Saturated fatty acids are usually solid at room temperature, and they're more stable than other types of fats — that is, they don't turn rancid as quickly.

Saturated fatty acids raise blood cholesterol, especially the LDL or "bad" cholesterol. Your risk of coronary heart disease rises as your blood cholesterol level increases.

The fat in meat is considered mostly saturated. You can see the visible fat of a piece of prime rib when it's served. You've probably noticed that when the juices that cook out of a roast start to cool, part of the fat starts to solidify and rise to the top. That fat that rises to the top is saturated fat. If you leave a stick of butter on the kitchen counter, it softens but doesn't become completely runny — that's because butter is saturated fat.

Trans fats are a subclass of saturated fat, but they started out as an unsaturated fat like vegetable oil. Food producers and snack makers *hydrogenated* (or added hydrogen to) the vegetable oils. Hydrogenated vegetable oils become more saturated and contain lots of trans fats. Hydrogenated vegetable oils are used in all kinds of common, everyday food products, such as fast food, French fries, stick margarine, and cookies.

In clinical studies, trans fatty acids, or hydrogenated fats, tend to raise total blood cholesterol levels more than unsaturated fats, but less than more-saturated fatty acids. Trans fatty acids also tend to raise LDL ("bad") cholesterol and lower HDL ("good") cholesterol. These changes in cholesterol levels may increase your risk of heart disease.

Saturated fats and trans fatty acids are the two major culprits that have given fat its nasty reputation. These two troublemakers are associated with a whole host of medical conditions including heart disease, arteriosclerosis, cancer, high blood pressure, and diabetes. However, with a few changes to your diet, you can reduce the bad (saturated and trans fat), but still keep the good (and necessary!) mono- and polyunsaturated fats.

Limiting saturated fats in your diet basically means avoiding high-fat red meats and whole-fat dairy products. Eliminating all the saturated fat in your diet isn't necessary. Eating saturated fats in the right proportion with unsaturated fats — at least 2 to 1 (unsaturated to saturated) — is perfectly fine. What that means for you is this:

- ✔ Reduce the saturated fat in your diet as much as possible and always eat at least twice as much unsaturated fat as you eat saturated.
- ✔ Eat only lean or extra-lean red meat.
- ✔ Only eat skim or very-low-fat dairy products.
- ✔ Eat more nuts and seeds.
- ✔ Try to eat fish two times per week.
- ✔ Use olive, canola, or peanut oils.
- ✔ Eat more olives and avocados.

Also avoid trans fat whenever and wherever you can. All vegetable shortenings are packed with trans fats. So are most brands of stick margarines. Some margarine makers are now offering brands that are low in saturated fat and are virtually free of trans fats. Examine labels carefully and look for "Contains 0 grams of trans fatty acids" on the label.

Keep in mind that at least 50 percent of the trans fats you eat are hidden in commercially baked goods (like crackers, muffins, and cookies), in other prepared foods, and in fried foods prepared in restaurants.

Monounsaturated fats

Monounsaturated oils are liquid at room temperature but start to solidify at refrigerator temperatures. This is why salad dressing containing olive oil turns cloudy when refrigerated but is clear at room temperature — olive oil is a monounsaturated fat. Likewise, the fat in natural peanut butter is mostly unsaturated. If you let a jar of natural peanut butter sit for a while, you'll notice an oily layer forms on the top. That liquid is peanut oil, which is unsaturated fat and a liquid at room temperature.

Monounsaturated fatty acids lower blood cholesterol. They lower the LDL ("bad") cholesterol, and increase the HDL ("good") cholesterol (which is a good thing). They also seem to lower triglycerides in some people when substituted for carbohydrate in the diet.

You can get your daily supply of monounsaturated fats from a variety of naturally occurring food sources including almonds, avocados, canola oil, cashews, olive oil, olives, peanut butter, peanut oil, peanuts, pecans, sesame seeds, and tahini paste made from sesame seeds.

Polyunsaturated fats

Polyunsaturated oils are liquid at room temperature and in the refrigerator. They easily combine with oxygen in the air to become rancid.

Polyunsaturated fatty acids help lower total blood cholesterol — by lowering the LDL ("bad") cholesterol but not the HDL ("good") cholesterol. The primary sources of polyunsaturated fat are margarine (the tub or squeeze kind, but not stick), English walnuts, corn oil, safflower oil, soybean oil, reduced-fat salad dressings, and mayonnaise.

Omega-3 fatty acids are a special class of polyunsaturated fatty acids found primarily in fish and fish oils but can also be found in flaxseed, walnuts, and soy and canola oils. Studies suggest these fatty acids may help reduce your risk of heart disease, stroke, and cancer. We know that omega-3 fatty acids lower LDL ("bad") cholesterol and triglycerides. Great sources of omega-3 fatty acids include salmon, albacore tuna, trout, herring, mackerel, flaxseeds, walnuts, canola oil, and non-hydrogenated soybean oil.

Omega-6 fatty acids are another class of polyunsaturated fatty acids. Linoleic acid comprises the majority of the polyunsaturated fat eaten in the United States and comes from a variety of commonly consumed animal and vegetable products, like corn, safflower, sunflower, and cottonseed oils.

In healthy populations that consume traditional diets, the ratio of omega-6 fat to omega-3 fat ranges from 5:1 to 10:1. In the American diet, the ratio is currently estimated to be 20:1. This imbalance is now potentially being linked to cancer, heart disease, and arthritis. Improving the ratio by substituting omega-3 fats for omega-6 fats in your diet could result in significant health benefits.

Finding trans fat on food labels

To help foods stay fresh on the shelf or to get a solid fat product, such as margarine, food manufacturers *hydrogenate* (or add hydrogen to) polyunsaturated oils. These fats are trans fats (covered earlier in this chapter), and you definitely want to avoid them. Trans fats increase LDL or "bad" cholesterol, and decrease HDL or "good" cholesterol, and raise triglycerides (another risk factor for heart disease). But how can you tell where they lurk? Products that list *partially hydrogenated vegetable oil* or *vegetable shortening* on the label are examples of trans fats.

Thanks to increased pressure from concerned consumers, dietitians, and other medical professionals, the Food and Drug Administration (FDA) will soon require listing of trans fats on the nutritional labels of all foods. Currently, the labels include total fat grams, polyunsaturated fat grams, saturated fat grams, and sometimes the voluntary listing of monounsaturated fat grams.

In July 2003, the FDA announced it would require food manufacturers to list trans fatty acids on the Nutrition Facts label. This additional information will give consumers a more complete picture of the fat content of foods. Some food products already list trans fat on the food label, but food manufacturers have until January 1, 2006, to comply.

Watch out for promises on products like "97-percent fat free." These messages may lead you to believe that if you eat a serving of this item, you'll only be getting 3 percent of the calories in fat grams. Not true! These types of statements reflect the percentage by *weight,* not by percentage of *calories.* The official FDA Nutrition Facts label is your best source for information on the true fat content of food.

Remember: Read the label! Products sold as healthy or cholesterol-free often contain vegetable oils that are so altered by processing that their inherent healthy properties have been stripped away.

Knowing How Much Fat Is Enough

One serving of fat contains 45 calories and 5 grams of fat. For the average healthy adult, eight fat servings per day are appropriate. And most of those servings (at least six) should be unsaturated fat. That means more avocados but less mayonnaise; more nuts and olives but fewer full-fat dairy products; more fish and poultry; and only lean red meats.

So how do you keep your fat intake on track? Try the following suggestions:

- ✔ Avoid saturated fat, which is animal fat found in red meat and full-fat dairy products, by eating lean meats, skim milk, and low-fat cheeses.

- ✔ Eat more nuts, legumes, poultry, and fish.

- ✔ Use nonstick cooking spray and liquid and spray margarine, soft tub margarines, and margarine blends with yogurt.

- ✔ Try the Olive Oil-Yogurt Spread recipe later in this chapter for an even better substitute for butter or margarine.

Check out Table 8-1 for guidelines on how much of the foods you eat constitutes a serving of fat.

Table 8-1	Fat Servings
Food	**Amount for 1 Serving**
Monounsaturated Fats	
Almonds	6
Avocado, medium	⅛ of an avocado
Canola oil	1 teaspoon
Cashews	6
Mixed nuts (50 percent peanuts)	6
Olive oil	1 teaspoon
Olives, black	8 large
Olives, green, stuffed	10 large
Peanut butter	2 teaspoons
Peanut oil	1 teaspoon
Peanuts	10
Pecans	4 halves
Sesame seeds	1 tablespoon
Tahini paste	2 teaspoons
Polyunsaturated Fats	
Corn oil	2 tablespoons
Margarine	1 teaspoon
Margarine, lower fat (30-percent to 50-percent vegetable oil, the rest water)	1 tablespoon
Mayonnaise, reduced-fat	1 tablespoon
Miracle Whip Salad Dressing, reduced-fat	1 tablespoon
Pumpkin seeds	1 tablespoon
Safflower oil	2 tablespoons
Soybean oil	2 tablespoons

(continued)

Table 8-1 *(continued)*

Food	Amount for 1 Serving
Polyunsaturated Fats	
Sunflower seeds	1 tablespoon
Walnuts, English	4 halves
Saturated Fat	
Bacon	1 slice
Butter, reduced-fat	1 tablespoon
Butter, stick	1 teaspoon
Butter, whipped	2 teaspoons
Cream, heavy, whipping	1 tablespoon
Cream, light or half-and-half	2 tablespoons
Cream cheese, reduced-fat	2 tablespoons
Cream cheese, regular	1 tablespoon
Neufchatel cheese	2 tablespoons
Salt pork	¼ ounce
Shortening or lard	1 teaspoon
Sour cream, reduced-fat	3 tablespoons
Sour cream, regular	2 tablespoons

Including More Healthy Fat in Your Diet

Replacing fats in the diet with refined carbohydrate creates new health problems; replacing saturated fat in the diet with unsaturated fat in the diet promotes better health. With a few simple changes, you can benefit from this proven diet plan.

Use liquid vegetable oils in cooking and at the table. Dipping bread in olive oil flavored with black pepper and coarse sea salt is a much better health choice than slathering it with butter. A little squeeze of liquid margarine is a better choice than pats of butter on steamed veggies.

Remember the calorie density of fat (9 calories per gram). Don't let fat dominate your food intake, but sneak good fats in. When making a salad, add sliced olives instead of cheddar cheese. Toss in some sliced almonds instead of bacon with your green beans. Don't increase your total fat intake, but do change the type of fat you eat.

Use olive oil as a replacement for the saturated fat in your diet. Olive oil makes all food more flavorful, fresh-tasting, and delicious. It's a natural choice for good health. Olive oil contains no cholesterol, chemicals, or artificial additives. It's especially high in monounsaturated fat, which may reduce harmful LDL cholesterol and help maintain healthy HDL cholesterol levels when substituted for saturated fat. Check out the recipes for the healthy spreads later in this chapter, and use them on salads, steamed veggies, fish and chicken, or that occasional bagel or cracker that's part of your carb count.

Try the following recipes for spreads. Olive oil makes them smooth and flavorful. They can be refrigerated for three or four days or frozen. Prepare them in advance for parties, special occasions, or just plain great snacking.

☞ *Yogurt–Olive Oil Spread or Base*

Preparation time: *15 minutes (plus 24 hours standing time)*

Cooking time: *None*

Yield: *12 ounces or about 1½ cups*

32-ounce container nonfat plain yogurt	*3 tablespoons olive oil*	*½ teaspoon salt (optional)*

1 Line a medium-size strainer with a coffee filter or a double layer of cheese cloth hanging over the rim. Suspend over a bowl to catch the *whey* (watery, liquid drippings that form). Spoon the yogurt into the prepared strainer and let stand, covered, for 24 hours in the refrigerator. It should yield about 20 ounces (1½ cups) drained yogurt. Reserve the whey for another use or discard it.

2 Place the drained yogurt in a mixing bowl. Slowly drizzle in the olive oil while stirring constantly until all the oil is incorporated. Add salt, if desired. Serve as is, or proceed with your recipe of choice. Store in the refrigerator for up to 1 week.

Note: *You can use this recipe as a spread or salad dressing; as a topping for steamed vegetables, grilled chicken, fish, or lamb; as a marinade for chicken, fish, or lamb; or as a dip for raw vegetables or fruit. Use the remaining liquid in soups, stews, sauces, and so on.*

Per 1 tablespoon: *Calories 32 (From Fat 15); Fat 2g (Saturated 0g); Cholesterol 1mg; Sodium 23mg; Carbohydrate 3g (Dietary Fiber 0g); Protein 2g.*

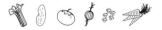

Cholesterol-reducing spreads

There are two new margarine-like products on the market — Benecol and Take Control — which are designed to lower cholesterol. You can find them in the dairy case next to butter and margarine. These products are made from plant sterol esters from canola or soybean oil. This new food ingredient can help reduce LDL cholesterol by blocking the absorption of cholesterol from the digestive tract. You need to eat two to three servings per day to reap the cholesterol-lowering benefit, however. For people with high cholesterol, these products can complement the effectiveness of their cholesterol-lowering medication.

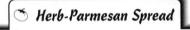 *Herb-Parmesan Spread*

Preparation time: *15 minutes (plus 1 hour standing time)*

Cooking time: *None*

Yield: *About 3 cups*

Yogurt–Olive Oil Spread or Base (see recipe earlier in this chapter)

¾ cup finely chopped green onion, white and green parts

½ cup grated Parmesan cheese

¼ teaspoon ground pepper

⅓ cup chopped flat-leaf parsley

Place the Yogurt-Olive Oil Spread or Base in a mixing bowl. Add the other ingredients, mix well, and let stand for 1 hour, allowing the flavors to marry. Serve as a spread on allowed crackers or melba toast, as a dip for raw vegetables, or as a topping for steamed vegetables.

Per 1 tablespoon: *Calories 20 (From Fat 10); Fat 1g (Saturated 0g); Cholesterol 1mg; Sodium 27mg; Carbohydrate 2g (Dietary Fiber 0g); Protein 1g.*

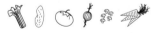

☞ Mushroom and Sun-Dried Tomato Spread

Preparation time: *15 minutes (plus 1 hour standing time)*

Cooking time: *None*

Yield: *1 cup*

2 cups chopped or sliced white button mushrooms	*½ teaspoon fresh thyme leaves or ¼ teaspoon dried thyme*
¼ cup chopped onion	*¼ teaspoon salt, or to taste*
4 tablespoons olive oil, divided	*Coarsely ground pepper to taste*
1 tablespoon chopped parsley	*1 tablespoon rinsed and drained, finely diced, oil packed sun-dried tomatoes*

1 In a skillet, combine the mushrooms, onion, and 1 tablespoon of the olive oil; cook until golden and until most of the liquid has evaporated; add the parsley, thyme, salt, and pepper.

2 In a food processor, puree the mushroom mixture. With the motor running, gradually add the remaining 3 tablespoons of olive oil through the feed tube. Transfer to a small bowl, and stir in the sun-dried tomatoes. Serve the spread on veggies or fruit slices, or on allowed crackers or melba rounds.

Per 1 tablespoon: Calories 34 (From Fat 31); Fat 4g (Saturated 1g); Cholesterol 0mg; Sodium 38mg; Carbohydrate 1g (Dietary Fiber 0g); Protein 0g.

Is butter better than margarine?

The potential cholesterol-raising effects of trans fatty acids have raised concern about the use of margarine and whether other options, including butter, may be better choices. Some stick margarines contribute more trans fatty acids than unhydrogenated oils or other fats.

Butter is rich in both saturated fat and cholesterol. That means it can cause the arteries to be blocked. Most margarine is made from vegetable fat and provides no dietary cholesterol. The more liquid the margarine (in tub or liquid form), the less hydrogenated it is and the fewer trans fatty acids it contains.

Improving Your Ratio of Good Fats to Bad Fats

Moderate, don't eliminate your fat intake. Mix up the kinds of fat you eat. Deliberately lower your saturated fat intake, but add more unsaturated fat, especially olive oil, peanut oil, canola oil, fish, olives, avocadoes, nuts, and nut oils. Eat two fish meals each week to increase your chances of getting omega-3 fatty acids in your diet.

Try to balance your intake of omega-3 and omega-6 fatty acids. Eat more fatty fish (salmon, albacore tuna, trout, herring, and mackerel), canola oil, flaxseed, and walnuts. Eat less corn, safflower, sunflower, and cottonseed oils.

Flaxseed contains high amounts of cancer fighters, as well as omega-3 fatty acids, which may help prevent heart disease. It also supplies iron, niacin, phosphorous, and vitamin E. To release the health benefits of flaxseed, the hard outer coating must be broken down. Place flaxseed in a small nonstick skillet; cook over low heat 5 minutes or until toasted, stirring constantly. Place the flaxseed in a blender; process just until chopped. Flaxseed keeps best when stored in the refrigerator. Toast and chop right before using.

Here are some other ways to improve your ratio of good fats to bad fats:

- **Try a few nuts for a snack.** But remember that 1 cup of nuts is about 800 calories, so don't eat too many!

- **Use thin slices of avocado in place of mayonnaise.**

- **Always use the reduced-fat version of a high-fat food.** For example, try reduced-fat mayonnaise, reduced-fat salad dressing, reduced-fat Miracle Whip, and reduced-fat cheeses.

- **Combine cheese with fruit to lower the fat percentage for the whole snack.**

- **Avoid trans fats whenever possible.** Watch for ingredients like partially hydrogenated fat. Choose tub over stick margarine. Avoid shortening, commercially prepared breads, pastries, cookies, and french fries.

Part III
Shopping, Cooking, and Dining Out

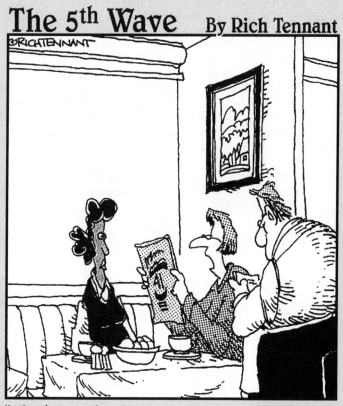

The 5th Wave   By Rich Tennant

"I'll have the 'Low-Carb-High-Fiber-Low-Fat-I'll-Just-Have-A-Bite-of-My Neighbor's-Eggs-Benedict-Breakfast'."

In this part . . .

I expand on the Whole Foods Eating Plan and get you started with planning your meals, shopping, and dining out, the low-carb way. I show you how to get in and out of the supermarket with low-carb foods — without gouging your wallet. I also reveal the mystery of food labels. I give you great suggestions for quick and easy breakfasts, grab-and-go lunches, and delicious dinners. You'll discover how to calculate carbohydrates in your favorite recipes and (I hope) find some new favorites. I've included some of my favorite low-carb comfort foods (really!) and sides and entrees perfect for entertaining. And how would any of us get along without eating out once in a while? I guide you through this tricky part of any dieting plan and give great suggestions for eating out in any scenario, including fast-food restaurants.

Chapter 9

Navigating the Supermarket

· ·

In This Chapter

▶ Discovering supermarket psychology

▶ Understanding supermarket layout

▶ Steering yourself toward healthy foods

▶ Deciphering food labels

· ·

*Y*ou're headed home and you decide to run into the supermarket to pick up milk and bread; you leave 20 minutes later with four bags of groceries. But don't blame yourself. From the time you entered the store, your behavior was controlled. Supermarkets are carefully planned to see that you leave the store with more than you came in for. Supermarket layout is an art and a science. Supermarkets are creatively and scientifically designed to enhance your spending. From the music that you hear, to the aromas that you smell, you need to be aware of the environment you're entering — not only to keep your spending down, but to avoid those impulse items that are not part of your healthy eating plan.

If it goes in the grocery cart, it goes in the house and it goes in the mouth. Stop and think before you toss something into your cart.

Understanding Supermarket Psychology

Most shoppers don't give a second thought to where the cereal or green beans sit on the store's shelves. But supermarket managers know that over 50 percent of purchases are bought on impulse. In many cases, representatives from food manufacturers work with supermarket managers to place their product lines on grocery store shelves. Depending on how well the products are arranged, they can boost profits or hurt sales.

Large supermarkets carry over 50,000 items on their shelves with thousands of new products appearing every year. The competition for *shelf space,* or space for items to be placed on the shelves, is fierce. Products sitting on shelves too long and taking up space are quickly replaced by better-selling items. The objective is to keep the product line moving.

The layout of the supermarket is designed to keep you in the store longer than you planned. Time is very critical. Every minute you spend browsing is another minute in which you're more likely to spend that extra dollar.

Even though products such as milk, bread, and meat are considered necessary commodities, you often find them at the back of the store, many times on opposite ends of the store. So, in your rush to pick up milk and bread, you will likely travel the entire length (and maybe width) of the store.

Try out this scenario: When you enter the store, you first reach for the hand basket because you say to yourself, "It's only a couple of items. I can manage." But then you remember how heavy that gallon of milk is when you carry it in that small basket back up to the cashier at the front of the store. So, you choose the grocery cart instead. You pick up your gallon of milk and, on your way to the bread display, the wonderful aroma of baking bread gets your attention. So you pick up the sandwich bread in the bread aisle you intended to buy and head for the bakery. Going back in front of the dairy case you noticed crocks of butter. You think, "Now, that'd be good on warm bread." Picking up the butter you proceed to the bakery. Passing the meat counter, you catch a whiff of barbequed roast. You think, "Well, it is close to dinnertime and I am feeling pretty hungry." That roast is fully prepared and ready to go. Placing it in your cart you head for the bakery. Slowing down for a minor traffic jam of grocery carts, you notice a bright display of canned baked beans marked "3 for $5." Picking up three cans, you head for the bakery. Arriving at the bakery, you're thinking, "Why am I here? Oh yeah, the bread."

Are you starting to get the picture? Store managers and food manufacturers got the picture a long time ago and have created ambience in grocery stores to encourage people to stay longer and longer. From the little café tables by the coffee vendor, to the familiar music they play, the longer you stay, the more you'll pay.

Knowing Supermarket Layout and Design

In this section, I show you how your grocery store layout and design affects your purchases. Check out Figure 9-1 for an illustration of a typical grocery store layout.

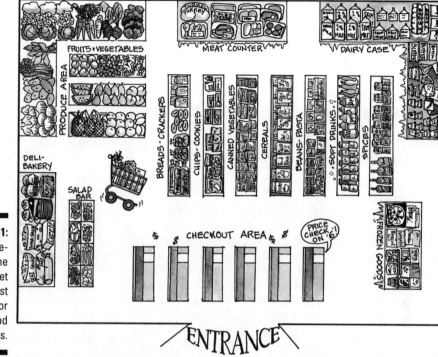

Figure 9-1:
The perimeter of the supermarket is your best bet for whole-food choices.

Patrolling the perimeter

The most basic and nutritious foods are usually placed in areas around the perimeter of the store. This is where you find milk, bread, meat, and produce. At least one of these staple items is on every shopping list. Locating them around the edge and toward the back of the store provides more opportunity for bright-colored displays to catch your eye.

Eyeing the endcaps

Located at the end of the aisles, these eye-catching displays generally showcase items the store wants to sell quickly. These items may or may not be sale-priced.

Hitting at eye level

Costly items with the highest profit margins for the store are generally placed on shelves at shoppers' eye level. Check above or below for better deals.

Targeting your child

Cereals with cartoon characters and free toys are placed at a child's eye level. Larger bags of candy and specialty toys are at a kid's eye level as well.

Anticipating traffic jams

Some interruption of grocery-cart travel is allowed to occur in order to slow you down and cause you to browse.

Seducing you with signs

So-called "specials" may only be special to the store. When you see something labeled as a special, that doesn't guarantee the item will have a lower price.

When you see something marked with "as advertised," you may think that the item is on sale. But these signs don't necessarily translate into sale-priced or even regularly well-priced items.

Another trick to get you to buy more is advertising "3 for $5" or something similar. But if the management is playing fair, you can get the special price buying just one of the items — you don't have to pick up three.

Heading into the holidays

Supermarkets make purchasing items for holiday celebrations easy. But have you noticed how early it starts? Right after Labor Day you'll see Halloween candy in the store. How many trick-or-treaters do you see in September? The holiday is two months away! Buying candy too soon creates temptation for you, which candy makers hope will make you buy twice as much (some to eat now, some to give away later).

Luring you with free samples

Those nice ladies encouraging you to sample their wares are demonstrating a highly successful selling technique. You wouldn't want to hurt their feelings by turning down their hospitality, would you? And if you're hungry when in the store, you may give in to tempting foods that end up in your cart.

Grooving to the music

Supermarket music is becoming synonymous with elevator music. The slow, lulling tempo encourages more browsing.

Steering Your Cart toward the Healthy Foods

Put the following locations on your radar screen as targets for healthy food:

- **Perimeter:** The healthiest foods are around the perimeter of the store. This is where you'll find the most *whole foods* — foods free from processing and added sugar, salt, and fat.

- **Dairy case:** Look for skim, ½%, and 1% milk; low-fat and nonfat yogurt; reduced-fat cheeses; ricotta cheese; and liquid or tub margarines labeled with "no trans fatty acids."

- **Produce section:** People study years to memorize all the carotenoids, flavonoids, antioxidants, phytochemicals, and other wonderful stuff in fruits and vegetables. And let's face it, you're probably not that interested in the science behind it all. So just concentrate on filling your cart with color. Get as many colors in there as possible — red, yellow, orange, and especially green — and you'll cover all the bases. Buy fruit in season and in bags. Apples and oranges sold in bags are often cheaper than purchasing the same fruits individually.

Here are a few tips to help you select the best produce.

- Choose produce with a good color, not pale or browning.

- Select firm, not limp or soggy, produce. Hard pieces are not yet ripe; soft pieces are too ripe. If you're making guacamole, select the mushiest avocados you can find — the riper the better.

- Avoid bruised or damaged items.

- Ask the produce manager if you can sample the food before buying. Nothing is more frustrating than getting home and discovering the grapes are sour.

- **Meat counter:** Don't fear red meat, but look for the leanest cuts available. Red meat is an important source of zinc and iron. Check out those lean suggestions in Chapter 5 and on the grocery list in Appendix C.

- **Fish market:** Get acquainted with your store's fish market. Fish is a heart-healthy food. The American Heart Association recommends two fish meals a week. Try the easy recipes located in Chapter 12.

It's best to purchase fresh fish the same day you plan to prepare it. If you don't do that, store fresh fish sandwiched between layers of ice (see Figure 9-2) or in airtight plastic containers. Don't purchase fish with a "fishy" odor.

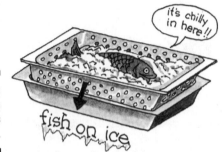

Figure 9-2:
Store fish
in layers
of ice.

Supermarket salad bars offer a convenient variety of already prepared fruits and vegetables — no cutting, no mess. Also, try prepackaged salads, greens, and slaws. Containers of cut-up fruit (pineapple rings, sliced strawberries, melon balls, kiwi slices, mango, and papaya chunks) can be eaten as is or mixed into cereal or frozen yogurt. You may pay a little more, but sometimes paying for this convenience results in a healthier meal at home than a trip to a fast-food restaurant.

Avoiding Pitfalls in the Aisles

The middle aisles are where all the processed foods are (refer to Figure 9-1). The more ingredients a food has that you can't pronounce, the less it belongs in your shopping cart. But there are some good choices in the aisles if you know where to look.

Here are a few examples of healthy foods that are found in the aisles, rather than at the perimeter of the grocery store:

- ✔ **Dried beans:** An inexpensive source of protein and fiber, dried beans and peas are a good way to spend one of your carbohydrate choices.

- ✔ **Peanut butter:** Not all peanut butters are created equal. The healthiest choices are those that contain only peanuts and salt. Some have trace amounts (less than 1 percent) of hydrogenated vegetable oils (trans fatty acids that threaten heart health) or corn syrup. The small amount of hydrogenated oil keeps the peanut butter from separating and makes the peanut butter creamier. Read food labels carefully.

✔ **Whole-grain bread:** Don't assume that breads with names like "whole-grain" are good sources of fiber. You must check the ingredient panel and look for the word *whole*. A *real* whole-grain bread will list "whole-grain wheat flour" as the first or second ingredient. Also, look for brands that contain at least 3 grams of fiber per serving.

✔ **Canned fruits:** Look for fruits canned in a light syrup or in their own juice. They're great to keep in the pantry to add to a meal. Check out the recipes in Chapters 11 and 12 for ways to use canned fruit. Avoid canned fruit juice products that aren't 100-percent juice, and seek out those that have been fortified with vitamin C and calcium. Look for fruit prepackaged in individual serving containers for quick lunchbox additions.

✔ **Canned vegetables:** Canned vegetables are better than no vegetables at all and in some cases may be better. Keep them in the pantry ready to add to a quick meal, salad, or soup.

Recent studies show that the phytochemicals known as *carotenoids* are better absorbed from many cooked, rather than raw, foods. Carotenoids are powerful antioxidants that are present in red, orange, and yellow vegetables and fruits. Lycopene, a phytochemical shown to fight cancer, becomes more available in tomato products that have been exposed to heat, such as canned or stewed tomatoes, pasta sauce, and ketchup. Carrots have higher levels of beta-carotene after cooking. Corn's antioxidant activity is increased the longer it is cooked. However, levels of folate (a B vitamin) and vitamin C can be decreased by cooking.

✔ **Canned soups:** Canned soups are notorious for being high in sodium and fat. Don't assume that just because a soup claims to be low in fat that it is also low in sodium. Look for soups with less than 500 mg of sodium and less than 3 grams of fat per serving.

✔ **Spaghetti sauce:** Like canned soups, spaghetti sauces differ in sodium content and fat content. Look for a sauce with fewer than 500 mg of sodium and 3 grams of fat per serving. Or try making your own spaghetti sauce using unseasoned canned tomato sauce and adding your own minced garlic and fresh basil. You can find brands of tomato sauce with as little as 0 grams of fat and 200 mg of sodium.

✔ **Frozen foods:** Frozen dinners can be a healthy choice if you carefully select them. Look for dinners that contain about 1 cup of vegetables and about 350 to 400 calories. Plan to add a salad, a piece of fruit, or a glass of skim milk to improve the nutritional quality and to make the meal more satisfying. Many frozen dinners are high in sodium and fat so look for dinners with no more than 800 mg of sodium and no more than 30 percent of the daily value for total fat. Keep a few frozen dinners in the freezer. They're perfect for a quick dinner when time is limited or when you just don't feel like cooking.

Frozen vegetables (without sauces) are just as nutritious as fresh. Buy the large-sized bags. Take out what you need and save the rest for later. You can add bags or boxes of frozen veggies to already prepared soups, stews, and casseroles.

What's the skinny on natural peanut butter?

You'll recognize natural peanut butter by the oily layer that forms on the top. Don't pour this oil off. It is a monounsaturated fat and good for your heart. Also, pouring it off will leave a very thick peanut butter that not only sticks to the roof of your mouth but is impossible to spread on bread. You can handle the oil in two ways:

✔ Just turn the jar over until the oil seeps through to the other end. Periodically rotate

the jar to keep the oil evenly dispersed in the peanut butter.

✔ Take a knife and carefully stir the oil back down into the peanut butter. When it's evenly mixed, store the peanut butter in the refrigerator to keep it from separating. When ready to use, take out the portion needed and soften it in the microwave for spreading.

Deciphering Food Labels

Always read the labels. Get out of the habit of only looking at the fat content. Look at the total carbohydrate content per serving. Determine how much is fiber and how much is sugar. Look at the ingredient list and determine the food sources of the fat, carbohydrate, and fiber. The more dietary fiber in the food the better it is.

If the food you're evaluating has a high carb count and it's mainly high fructose corn syrup or table sugar, remember that 4 grams of sugar equal 1 teaspoon. Regular 12-ounce cans of soft drink contain 40 grams of carbohydrate — all sugar. That equals 10 teaspoons, or almost ¼ cup. It's a sobering thought.

Check out the serving sizes. All the nutrition information on the label applies to the stated serving size. Don't assume that a small box of any food or beverage is only one serving. Double-check the number of servings per container. Often a 16-ounce bottle contains 2 servings. But who only drinks half a bottle? You may be getting twice the sugar you thought.

Understanding the ingredient panel

Foods listed in the ingredient panel are required to be listed greatest in quantity (by weight) first and then on down the line. A breakfast cereal with sugar listed as first or second on the ingredient panel has more sugar than anything else.

Look for the terms _hydrogenized_ or _partially hydrogenated oil_ on the ingredient panel. This indicates a source of trans fatty acids. Try to minimize your intake of this fat. You'll find it in many packaged goods, such as cakes, pastries, crackers, cookies, and cereals. For more on trans fats, see Chapter 8.

Fresh produce does not carry a nutrition label. However, the nutrition information should be available. Look for it on a flyer or poster in the produce department. Ask the produce manager if you can't find it.

Discovering the Nutrition Facts label

The Nutrition Facts label issued by the Food and Drug Administration (FDA) in 1994 provides nutrition information relevant to current public health recommendations (see Figure 9-3). Its intent is to show how a food fits into an overall healthy diet. The label carries information that consumers can apply to their individual health needs.

Nutrition Facts
Serving Size 1/2 cup (122 g)
Servings Per Container about 3.5

Amount Per Serving

Calories 40   Fat Cal. 5

% Daily Value*

Total Fat 0.5 g	1%
Sodium 5 mg	0%
Total Carb. 9 g	3%
Fiber 5 g	21%
Sugars 4 g	
Protein 2 g	

Vitamin A 300% (80% as beta-carotene)

Calcium 2%   Iron 4%

Not a significant source of saturated fat, cholesterol, and vitamin C.
*Percent Daily Values are based on a 2,000 calorie diet.

Figure 9-3:
The
Nutrition
Facts label.

Serving size: This varies from package to package. Serving sizes don't always reflect the typical amount that an adult may eat. In some cases, the serving size may be a very small amount.

Calories: The calories contained in a single serving.

% daily values: The percentage of nutrients that one serving contributes to a 2,000-calorie diet. Parents or children may need more or less than 2,000 calories per day.

Nutrient amounts: The nutritional values of the most important, but not all, vitamins and other nutrients in the product.

The top section gives you information on the serving size of the food, and how many servings are in the entire container. The middle section of the label gives you details on the nutrients most important to good health. This section helps you to calculate daily limits for fat, cholesterol, sodium, carbohydrate, fiber, and other nutrients. Pay close attention to two things in this section:

✔ **Daily Reference Values (DRVs)** are standards for nutrients that have a significant impact on health and disease. DRVs for fat, saturated fat, carbohydrate, fiber, and protein are based on a 2,000-calorie reference diet. The 2,000-calorie level was chosen because it represents a reasonable reference caloric intake for an adult or for children over 4 years of age.

✔ **Percent (%) Daily Value:** The % Daily Value shows you how a food fits into your overall diet. If you see that a food contains 200 mg of cholesterol, you may not know if it is high or low in cholesterol. The % Daily Value is the clue. It tells you that one serving of the food has 66 percent of your daily value for cholesterol. A neat trick to use is to remember the 5 and 20 rule: If a food has 5% or less of a nutrient, it is considered low in that nutrient; if it has 20% or more, it's considered high.

Prior to the Nutrition Labeling and Education Act, many descriptive terms used on labels were not regulated. Today, food products using descriptive terms on food labels must meet strict regulations.

Nutrient content claims are defined for *one serving*. For example, that means that low-fat cheese has no more than 3 grams of fat per serving.

Considering labels on the Whole Foods Eating Plan

For the Whole Foods Eating Plan, you don't count the carbohydrate in fruits, vegetables, and milk. You only count the carbohydrate in the Yellow Light starchy foods. (See Chapter 6 for the full story.) Fruits, vegetables, and milk will show sugar as part of the total carbohydrate on the food label, but this sugar is the naturally occurring sugar in the food. It is not added sugar.

In the Yellow Light foods, 15 grams of total carbohydrate count as one carbohydrate choice. You may subtract the fiber from the total carbohydrate amount. For example, if one serving of a cereal contains 21 grams of total carbohydrate and 6 grams of dietary fiber, you may subtract the 6 grams of fiber from the total of 21 grams of carbohydrate. This will give you 15 grams of total carbohydrate for one serving, which equals one carb choice.

Be familiar with all the names in the ingredient list that mean sugar. For the sweet, or not-so-sweet, story on sugar, see Chapter 3.

Chapter 10

Planning Menus and Meals

In This Chapter

▶ Putting it all together

▶ Planning meals to please the whole family

▶ Entertaining guests the low-carb way

▶ Snacking between meals, with low-carb treats

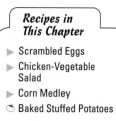

*Y*ou're headed home from work, starting to relax, and then it hits you: What's for dinner? You picture hungry mouths meeting you at the door, and you hear your own stomach starting to rumble. Panic-time! Everyone is waiting for you, they're starving, and you don't have enough time to cook something. Then you see it, as if it were divinely placed in your view to answer your problem: golden arches gleaming in the setting sun. Your car turns as if drawn by a magnet. In no time, you've pulled into your driveway and opened the door laden with sustenance as if you're back from the hunt with the fattest beast. Cheers greet you and, for a brief moment, you are the family hero.

Sound familiar? Whether it was McDonald's, KFC, or Pizza Hut that allowed you to be king or queen for a brief moment, that glory soon fades and the guilt sets in. You remember your last visit to the doctor and the warning of increasing cholesterol. Your spouse never has any energy and sleeps all the time. And the kids are looking a little pudgy.

I have good news: Sensible lower-carb eating will make you and your family feel great and will give you the energy to enjoy busy days. But it doesn't come naturally in today's environment. It requires thoughtful planning. In this chapter, I give you all the information you need to plan low-carb meals and resist the fast-food temptation.

Planning Menus Ahead

Low-carb eating can quickly become a way of life. You'll be amazed at your heightened energy level that comes with reducing the amount and improving the quality of carbohydrate in your diet. Using complex carbs to help sustain you helps you avoid sugar highs and lows, keeping you fuller longer and keeping energy levels constant. With dedicated low-carb dieting, you'll also lose unwanted pounds. Notice I said *dedicated* dieting. One key ingredient in the recipe for low-carb dieting is planning. The better prepared you are to handle the unexpected obstacles that your busy life throws your way, the more successful you'll be and the sooner you'll achieve your desired results.

Failing to plan is planning to fail

A wise plan of food selection can be the key to many happy, healthy years. Do people like to plan their eating? No, not really. If you're like most people, you're used to eating as a natural response to hunger or tempting foods. It's a mindless activity. And no one knows that better than marketers of snacks, sodas, and fast food. They like to make your eating decisions for you. Reaching for a pre-packaged snack is always easier than creating your own healthy item when you're hungry. So plan your snacks *before* you're hungry.

Should you plan your eating? Most certainly, at least until choosing healthy foods becomes automatic. You plan other important aspects of your life. Just as you plan other important events in your life, plan your eating. Why plan? To ensure success.

Developing your food-plan strategy

If you know that you have ballet lessons, soccer practice, or Cub Scouts on a particular night of the week, you can plan meals ahead of time rather than visit your local fast-food restaurant. If you know you'll be working late this week, make dinner ahead of time and freeze it for a healthy reheated meal. And you might consider just keeping a few things handy and ready in the freezer for those unexpected busy nights. Your strategy is as unique as your lifestyle. For more on examining your lifestyle with low-carb dieting in mind, check out Chapter 4.

Regardless of your lifestyle, these tips are helpful. Pick and choose your favorites.

- ✔ **Go grocery shopping only once a week.** With supermarkets so handy (and many open 24 hours a day), limiting your shopping to once a week isn't always easy to do, but it certainly cuts down on impulse buying. In addition, it saves you time and will encourage you to at least roughly plan your daily menus instead of just grabbing whatever's handy.

- ✔ **Cook in quantity.** Instead of one entree, make two. Enjoy one right away and freeze the other one to use later. Soups, spaghetti sauce, meat, and poultry dishes freeze well, so keep one of these in your freezer for when you don't feel like cooking. You can even freeze leftovers in individual serving containers. These containers are particularly handy for quick healthy frozen lunches.

✔ **Prepare larger cuts of meat like a roast, whole chicken, or a turkey breast.** It's a great way to provide several family meals but cook only once. Talk about tasty sandwiches and delicious lunchbox foods!

✔ **Have a marathon cooking session during the weekend.** If you're chopping onions for soup, you might as well keep chopping for spaghetti sauce. And since you're cooking in volume, you can definitely justify the cleanup of time-saving equipment like food processors. Cook and freeze for the week. This not only helps control the foods you consume, but cooking for the rest of the week is a breeze — and think of the cleanup saving! What a great stress relief!

✔ **Write it down!** Keep a food journal, especially keeping track of your carb choices. You can review it at the end of every day to make sure you're getting enough whole grains and legumes *and* not exceeding your daily carbohydrate choices.

Work on your own food strategy and spend some time with the Whole Foods Eating Plan:

✔ **Review the Green Light Foods in Chapter 5.** Mark the ones you really like and the ones you're willing to try. Add a new food to your grocery list every week.

✔ **Check out the Yellow Light list of starchy carbs in Chapter 6.** Select the ones to use and get to know the appropriate portion sizes.

✔ **Stock up on skim milk instead of whole milk and 2 percent.**

✔ **Start replacing saturated fats with unsaturated fats.** Switch to soft tub margarine rather than butter or stick margarine. Replace full-fat cheeses with crunchy nuts in your salads.

✔ **Keep lean meats on hand for quick entrees and snacks.** A rolled up piece of lean deli turkey is a great snack, right out of the package.

Scheduling for special occasions

We're conditioned to celebrate with food. Baby showers, birthday parties, wedding receptions, and many other occasions call for special, and often carb-heavy foods. If you know you have a special occasion on a particular day, compensate by adjusting your carbohydrate intake the rest of the day. That doesn't mean you should starve yourself all day because you're going to indulge in a big dinner.

Take advantage of the Green Light list in Chapter 5 and continue to eat through the day. Save your carb choices for a glass of wine or piece of cake.

Look for Green Light foods on the buffet. Veggie trays are a great place to find free foods. Be sure to watch the dips and count milk and carb choices as needed. Cocktail shrimp are definite Green Light foods. Meat and cheese trays can be a lifesaver if you're looking for a quick bite.

If you must turn your meat and cheese into a sandwich, choose the darkest, grainiest bread available. Without a food label handy, you won't be able to ensure that you have a whole-grain choice, but it's the most likely candidate. Also, choose mustard rather than mayo, unless it's clearly marked as reduced-fat.

Avoid the fried items like chicken wings or egg rolls. One egg-roll wrapper has 12 to 13 grams of carbs, and that doesn't even count the filling or dipping sauce! If they're just too tempting to avoid, make sure you count them with the appropriate carb choice.

The bottom line: Save your carb choices for the occasion, and make them count. Don't consume unwanted carbs in sugary marinades, like barbecue sauce or prepackaged chips and dips. Go for the most unrefined, natural food choices available at your event. And make sure you count your carb choices.

You have five carb choices to use every day — at least three of them should be whole-grain choices. Each carb serving is made up of around 15 grams of carbs. Check out Chapter 6 for serving sizes of your favorite foods.

Getting Organized

Any plan is only as good as its execution, and executing your plan is much easier if you're organized and ready. Here are a few easy tips that will get you ready to go in no time.

- ✔ **Arrange your pantry and freezer with foods sorted by their Whole Foods Eating Plan color, like Green Light on one shelf, Yellow Light on another, and so on.** This strategy makes it easy to grab ingredients that fit your needs. You can also take a quick visual inventory of what you have and don't have on grocery-shopping day.

- ✔ **Stock your pantry, refrigerator, and freezer with easy-to-fix, low-carb-friendly foods, such as canned and frozen vegetables, lean meats, fish fillets, and chicken.** Look for individually quick-frozen proteins, so you can thaw only what you need. You can find large bags of these individual chicken breasts at grocery stores and warehouse stores, so you can still save money and make small portions. Also, there's little to no waste with these trimmed prepared proteins. The fish portions are usually ready to use right out of the bag, no messy bones or skin to mess with. You can find frozen shrimp in a variety of forms — cooked, raw, or with or without shells. You can find individual beef burgers and chicken burgers for easy weeknight dinners.

✔ **Enlist members of your family to help with the planning.** Make the planning process a game using your recipe cards. Spread a few low-carb-friendly recipes out, face down on the table. Take turns picking up cards to create the weekly menu. Post the menu on the fridge, bulletin board, or chalkboard — wherever everyone is likely to see it. That way, whoever is home first knows what's for dinner and can start cooking.

✔ **Make friends with your microwave.** Microwave ovens are great for vegetables. They usually save time, retain nutrients, and maximize the natural flavor of vegetables. To get started, try Microwave Zucchini in Chapter 12. Or cook an entire ear of corn (husk and all) in the microwave, three minutes per ear. Remove the husk before eating, though, because no one needs *that* much fiber. Microwaving is also great for heating leftover vegetables. Try microwave or quick stovetop versions of dishes you usually bake.

Always pay attention to standing times in microwave recipes. Because microwave ovens can heat unevenly, these standing times give your dish a chance to even out temperature-wise.

✔ **Use other labor-saving devices, such as a food processor, convection oven, pressure cooker, slow cooker, or indoor grill.** Any cut of meat becomes tastier when stewed in a slow cooker. Dried beans, peas, and lentils are a snap to prepare quickly with a pressure cooker. The more you use a food processor, the more you'll wonder how you ever got along without it — especially if you cook in volume. You can dice 10 pounds of onions without shedding a single tear.

Maintaining grocery lists

Keep a running shopping list so you can jot down needed items as you think of them. Post your list in a conspicuous place, like on the fridge, and keep a pencil handy. Invite all family members to add to the list letting them know there may be substitutions for high-calorie, high-carbohydrate foods. To get started, take a look at the form in Appendix C. It lists all the foods in the book, and puts them in their appropriate categories. I've given you some extra spaces to fill in other items I've left off. Make copies of this great list and take one with you to the market — you'll always have a reminder of the best choices for your low-carb lifestyle.

Use your weekly menu to finish up your grocery list. It doesn't do much good to create a menu and advertise it for the family to see, only to find you don't have the items in the house to create your low-carb delights. Make sure that if you're going to have Jim's Sausage Soup (see Chapter 12 for details), you have Healthy Choice small link sausages on your list. An extra trip to the grocery store means more opportunity for impulse buying. Also, note any unusual quantities that you might need, so if you're making a double batch of Marilyn's Orange Pineapple Delight from Chapter 5, you'll have the necessary two 11-ounce cans of mandarin oranges.

Take your grocery list to the store on your weekly visit. All your hard work and planning is out the window if your list stays stuck to the fridge. Even though you may be able to avoid impulse buys, you're likely to make it home without that one secret ingredient for your Aunt Bunny's beef stew that you've painstakingly converted to a new low-carb entrée. For details on converting your own recipes, see Chapter 12.

If you're a budget-conscious shopper, take time to cross-reference your grocery list with the weekly grocery sales circular from the newspaper. You can make a notation by each of your items regarding which store has the best deals, saving you time and money.

Creating a snack list

Snacks are a necessary (and delicious!) part of healthy, low-carb dieting. Gone are the days of the nutrition advice, "Three square meals a day, and no in-between meal snacks." Instead, I recommend *preventive eating,* meaning eating healthy foods before you're hungry, to stave off hunger and eliminate the urge to overeat high-carb, prepackaged snacks.

Preventive eating is eating in order *not* to eat. In other words, use your Green Light foods to strategically place snacks in your day to help control your appetite at meals. Strategic times are mid-morning, mid-afternoon, arrival at home before dinner, or at bedtime. Other critical times include before a party or restaurant meal when you know you'll be tempted by high-calorie foods. Use only your Green Light foods for this purpose. Look for suggestions in the "Snacking the Good-Carb Way" section, later in this chapter. Any recipe in this book marked with a Green Light is a great snacking choice. Check out Chapters 11 and 12 for lots of great recipes.

Be sure to include room in your weekly menu and grocery list for preplanned snacks. Here are a few suggestions for your own snack list to get you started:

- An orange
- A bunch of grapes
- An 8-ounce container of low-fat yogurt
- A can of unsweetened applesauce, diced peaches, or mixed fruit
- A glass of skim, ½-percent, or 1-percent milk
- Dried apricots
- A handful of raisins
- A big green (or red) apple

- ✔ Raw vegetables (baby carrots, cherry tomatoes, green beans, pepper strips, radishes, celery, cucumber) with a low-fat salad dressing

- ✔ Sliced turkey rolled up in a lettuce leaf

- ✔ Boiled shrimp with zesty cocktail sauce

- ✔ Skim-milk mozzarella string cheese

Yellow Light foods make appropriate snacks on occasion, but you must plan for them and count them in your daily carbohydrate totals. Here are a few one-carb choice examples:

- ✔ 3 cups of low-fat microwave popcorn

- ✔ 1½ ounces of barbecued soy nuts

- ✔ Yogurt smoothie (see Chapter 12 for my Four-Fruit Shake)

Keep a chalkboard in the kitchen listing the snacks you have on hand. Kids think it's fun because it feels like a snack-bar menu, and it's handy because you don't have to hunt through the produce drawer. They can choose from fresh grapes, homemade granola, jicama chips, or sliced oranges. Just advertise the healthy choices that are your family's daily specials and reinforce good habits for the whole family. When you run out of one snack, just erase it or replace it with another.

Breakfast Quick and Easy

Breakfast is a meal that is often neglected and surrounded with excuses. Like, "I don't like bacon and eggs, and cereal makes me gag in the morning!", "I'm way too rushed in the morning, so I don't have enough time to eat," "I'm really not hungry when I first wake up," or, "I'm trying to lose weight, so I'll just save those calories."

None of those excuses are valid. The word *breakfast* comes from the phrase "break the fast." Our time of sleep is not only a time for rest and restoration, it's also the longest time most of us go in a 24-hour period without eating. The overnight fast from dinner until you wake up depletes the glucose stores necessary to keep your brain alert. During sleep, your metabolism drops to a maintenance level. A well-balanced morning meal ignites your mind and muscles for the day. It's like stoking the furnace or adding fresh wood to the dwindling campfire. Research demonstrates that skipping breakfast lowers mental performance especially in youth and young adults.

But analyze those excuses for a minute:

- **"I don't like traditional breakfast foods."** Who says breakfast has to be bacon and eggs, cereal and milk, or pancakes and syrup? Even left-over veggie or cheese pizza, or a peanut butter sandwich with orange juice can make a good breakfast. Just about any food can be a breakfast food, but there are a few exceptions. Avoid breakfasts high in refined carbohydrates or sugars. Sugary cereals, doughnuts, pastries, or pancakes and syrup may provide an immediate energy boost, but later in the morning you're more likely to be hungry and sleepy.

  Breakfast is a good time to use one or two of your less sweet and high-fiber carb choices. Carbohydrates are necessary to provide energy. Be sure to add a lean protein or a low-fat dairy food with it to provide additional energy and to keep you feeling "full." Fiber-rich whole-grain foods can also add to the feeling of fullness.

- **"My mornings are too hectic. There's just not enough time."** Plan ahead and stock the fridge with grab-and-go breakfasts. Whether you eat your breakfast in your kitchen, take it with you, or keep breakfast on hand at the office, it's faster than the drive-thru and a lot healthier. You can get a quick metabolism boost, by following a few easy tips:

  - Try setting out your breakfast the night before or getting ingredients together in the refrigerator. If you'd like a breakfast omelet, just do your prep the night before. Chop veggies, grate cheese, cook your bacon, and store it in the fridge. In the morning, you can break an egg or two and get going.

  - Stock your desk with non-perishable foods, such as packages of instant oatmeal, snack packs of raisins or other dried fruit, snack packs of nuts, small cans of 100-percent fruit juice or fruit canned in light syrup, jars of dried beef, or small tubs of applesauce or beef jerky.

  - Bring resealable plastic bags with premeasured portions of granola or other high-fiber cereal. Some vending machines in offices now carry both cereal and milk, and occasionally there are some whole-grain choices available. But don't count on it. Bring your own to ensure you can stay on your plan and hit your goals.

  - Keep packages of cheese and crackers or peanut butter and crackers to combine with a small can of fruit.

  - If you have a refrigerator at work, keep yogurt, low-fat cheese, skim milk, or fresh fruit. Be sure to count your carbs appropriately.

  - Buy a bigger lunchbox. Pack your breakfast — and your lunch — the night before.

- **"I'm not hungry in the morning."** An early work schedule or just concentrating on getting ready for the day make it difficult for some people to get in the mood to eat breakfast. But inevitably, hunger appears later in the morning. Don't be tempted by the pastry cart, lunch wagon, or vending machine. Before you leave the house, try starting off with something small like cheese and crackers or cottage cheese and fruit. At least drink some milk or juice before heading out. Then later in the morning, eat something more substantial like a whole-wheat muffin and a handful of grapes.

✔ **"I'm trying to lose weight, so I want to save my breakfast calories."** So you think skipping breakfast translates into automatic weight loss? Missing an entire meal would seem to eliminate a great deal of calories; however, when that meal is in the morning it can lead to bad habits like eating more high-calorie snacks and meals later on. Skipping breakfast leads to intense hunger, which makes it more difficult to make wise food choices. Eating breakfast jump-starts your metabolism and gets you started burning more calories, earlier in the day. Even just a quick container of low-fat or non-fat yogurt, a piece of fruit, or an ounce of low-fat cheese can get your calorie clock started.

Breakfast can energize you, maximize your mental potential, and keep your dietary intake on track. Start today developing your personal breakfast strategy.

Waking up fresh and healthy

Choose your main dish — whether it's cereal and milk, an egg, or a lean meat dish. If the dish is hearty, like hot cereal for example, you may want to serve a refreshing fruit juice with it. On the other hand, if it's less filling, a fruit combination or spiced fruit might lend an exciting contrast.

Check out a few ideas for easy breakfast menus.

Wake-up #1

Here's an easy family breakfast to get your day started right.

✔ Sparkling Fresh Fruit Cups (see Chapter 11 for recipe)

✔ Scrambled Eggs (recipe follows)

✔ Multigrain toast (counts as one carb choice)

✔ Soft tub margarine

✔ Skim milk, coffee, or tea

Scrambled Eggs

If you like super-fluffy scrambled eggs, try substituting water for the milk in this recipe. The water steams the eggs from the inside causing them to be lighter and fluffier. Delicious!

Preparation Time: 5 minutes

Cooking Time: 5 minutes

Yield: 3 servings

4 eggs

¼ cup skim milk

¼ teaspoon salt

Dash of pepper

Nonstick cooking spray

1 In small bowl, combine the eggs, milk, and seasonings. Heat a skillet over medium or medium-high heat.

2 Spray the heated skillet with nonstick cooking spray. Immediately, pour the eggs into a frying pan and stir from the outside edge toward the center, allowing the uncooked egg in the center to flow to the outside. Continue stirring until all the egg has cooked solid and has a creamy golden yellow appearance.

Vary It! Be creative and add chopped lean ham, chopped bell peppers and onions, or chopped mushrooms. Serve with picante sauce for a spicy flair.

Per serving: Calories 107 (From Fat 61); Fat 7g (Saturated 2g); Cholesterol 284mg; Sodium 288mg; Carbohydrate 2g (Dietary Fiber 0g); Protein 9g.

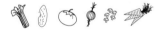

Wake-up #2

The beauty of this menu is that it can all be done ahead of time — great for families that start their morning on different time schedules. If you think brie is not the best choice for a morning cheese, consider substituting your family's favorite, like low-fat Monterey Jack, Colby, or cheddar.

- ✔ Fruit and Brie Kabobs (see Chapter 11 for recipe)
- ✔ Hearty Whole-Wheat Muffins (see Chapter 12 for recipe)
- ✔ Broiled Canadian bacon
- ✔ Skim milk, coffee, or tea

Make sure you count your muffin as one carbohydrate choice.

Wake-up #3

Perfect on a cold morning! This is the breakfast childhood was based on. I recommend that you use quick-cooking oats for a fast and easy weekday breakfast. Instant oatmeal can be a good choice — just watch how much sugar is added. Compare the nutrition labels of several varieties and watch the fiber stay constant while the overall carb count varies. That variation has to do with the amount of refined sugar the manufacturer adds.

- 100-percent orange juice
- Hot oatmeal
- Raisins or other dried fruit for topping
- Soft tub margarine (such as Brummel and Brown)
- Honey, brown sugar, or non-calorie sweeteners (optional)
- Broiled reduced-fat sausage patties
- Skim milk, coffee, or tea

Drink only 100-percent fruit juice. Juice drinks and punch are loaded with extra sugar and calories.

Grab-and-go breakfasts

Grab-and-go breakfasts are easy breakfasts that require little to no cooking and boast very easy cleanup, like yogurt topped with granola or berries or toast topped with eggs prepared in any fashion.

Try keeping a few things on this list handy in your fridge or pantry so you can grab and go in a hurry:

- Hard-boiled eggs or deviled eggs
- Small containers of 100-percent fruit juice
- Small containers of fruit packed in light syrup
- String cheese and whole-wheat crackers
- Veggies and low-fat dip
- Peanut butter and celery sticks

I hard-boil several eggs at once, usually six or so, to save time later on. Believe it or not, there are many ways to boil eggs. Here's my favorite method:

1. **Place a few eggs in a small saucepan.**

2. **Cover the eggs with water.**

   Make sure there's at least ½ inch of water over the eggs.

3. **Bring the water to a rolling boil and continue to boil for approximately 7 minutes.**

4. **Turn the water off, and allow the eggs to sit in the hot water for 10 minutes or so.**

5. **Run cool water over the eggs.**

6. **Peel and eat, or store unpeeled eggs in the fridge for up to one week.**

Grab-and-go breakfast #1

I like to sprinkle some of the granola into my yogurt to add a little crunch. You can portion out the granola in a resealable plastic bag the night before for extra speed.

- ✔ 1 container of low-fat fruit-flavored yogurt
- ✔ ½ cup Homemade Granola (see Chapter 12 for recipe)
- ✔ 1 small can of 100-percent fruit juice

Grab-and-go breakfast #2

String cheese is great to keep on hand. It stars in this delicious breakfast suggestion.

- ✔ 1 small can of 100-percent fruit juice
- ✔ 1 Fiber-Friendly Muffin (see Chapter 12 for recipe)
- ✔ 1 package of string cheese

Making Power Lunches

Lunch is the midday break for refueling, relaxing, and refreshing. Wherever you are — at home, the office, school, or a restaurant — take time to sit down and enjoy the food you're eating. Take a breather from whatever occupied the morning and restore your mental and physical energies for the afternoon's activities. Avoid heavy, high-carb meals. They will only leave you lethargic and sleepy at that after-lunch conference.

Noontime fuel

Use your lunchtime as a pit stop to power-up with Green Light foods and carbs low in glycemic load. For more on Green Light foods, see Chapter 5.

Because lunchtime is a time to refuel for the day, it's another good place to use one or two of your carbohydrate choices. I've put together a couple of tasty power lunches to get you through your day. As always, count your carb choices appropriately and if you find yourself still a bit hungrier, choose a food from the Green Light list.

Noontime fuel #1

This lunch requires a little work ahead of time, but it's well worth the effort. Share this lunch with special friends.

- ✔ Artichoke-Ham Bites (see Chapter 11 for recipe)
- ✔ Tasty Chicken Roll-Ups (see Chapter 11 for recipe)
- ✔ Steamy tomato soup
- ✔ Stone-ground whole-wheat thin crackers
- ✔ Frosty Fruit Cup (see Chapter 11 for recipe)
- ✔ Tea or coffee

If you eat one serving of each item on this menu, count it as a total of two carb choices. Seven roll-ups equal one carb choice and 14 crackers equal one carb choice.

Noontime fuel #2

This filling salad makes the meal! You won't believe you're dieting. If you're making it for a group, try using several different kinds of beans, like pinto, black beans, and cannellini beans.

- ✔ South of the Border Salad (see Chapter 12 for recipe)
- ✔ Light ranch salad dressing
- ✔ Blue Corn Crackers (see Chapter 12 for recipe)
- ✔ Light vanilla ice cream with fresh strawberries
- ✔ Tea or coffee

This salad has lots of Green Light foods, but make sure you count your carb choices. Seven crackers and the equivalent of ½ cup of beans in the salad count as one carb choice each for a total of two. If you also indulge in dessert, count your ½ cup scoop of ice cream as one dairy choice.

Noontime fuel #3

This lunch is almost too decadent to fall into the simple "fuel" category. It's a great choice for a leisurely weekend lunch when you have some extra time to linger over your cupcake and coffee.

- ✔ Tossed green salad ready-mix
- ✔ Lo-Cal Salad Dressing (see Chapter 12 for recipe)
- ✔ Onion-Lemon Fish with Quick Dill Sauce (see Chapter 12 for recipe)
- ✔ Summer Squash Medley (see Chapter 12 for recipe)
- ✔ Oat-Bran Bread (see Chapter 12 for recipe)
- ✔ Peanutty Cupcakes (see Chapter 11 for recipe)
- ✔ Tea or coffee

You won't even mind counting these carbohydrate choices. For each 1½-inch slice of Oat-Bran Bread, count one carb choice. One cupcake will cost you one carb choice — and you won't even ask for change.

Brown-bag bounty

Start viewing taking your lunch as a positive thing! It keeps you from standing in the fast-food line (or sitting in the drive-thru), eating out of the vending machine (at astronomical prices), or going out for a heavier lunch than you planned. It also gives you complete control over portion sizes. Be creative when making that sandwich, and vary the menu by taking a salad or left-over foods from home. Choose foods ahead of time that fit your individual meal plan.

Be wary when shopping for lunch items at the grocery store. Use processed foods and prepackaged products, like frozen entrées, sparingly. They tend to be overloaded with carbs, fat, preservatives, sugar, and sodium.

As with most rules, there are always exceptions, so look for these individually portioned foods to make brown-bagging a breeze *and* low-carb friendly:

- ✔ Unsweetened applesauce
- ✔ Canned fruits in their own juice
- ✔ Cans of tomato or vegetable juice
- ✔ Beef jerky
- ✔ Sugar-free and fat-free pudding and gelatin
- ✔ Low-fat or fat-free yogurt

✔ String cheese

✔ Peanut butter and cheese crackers

✔ Fruit-filled cereal bars

Brown-bag bounty #1

This is a basic sack lunch, but it's a welcome treat when the clock strikes twelve!

Package the lettuce and sliced tomatoes separately and add them to your sandwich before eating — this keeps your bread from getting soggy and keeps your lettuce crisp!

✔ Baby carrots with low-fat dip

✔ Ham-and-cheese sandwich made with:

- • 2 slices whole-wheat, 40-calorie bread

- • Thin-sliced Swiss cheese

- • Thin-sliced lean honey ham

- • Lettuce leaves and sliced tomatoes

- • Reduced-fat mayonnaise and spicy mustard (optional)

✔ Dill pickle

✔ Apple wedges with Apple-Cheese Spread (see Chapter11 for recipe)

✔ Diet soda or a bottle of sparkling water

If you're using the 40-calorie-per-slice whole-wheat bread, count two slices as one carb choice. Two pieces of any other bread will likely cost you two carb choices — check your food labels to be sure. Go whole grains!

Brown-bag bounty #2

Make this chicken salad the night before to save time in the morning. Sometimes I skip the crackers and eat my chicken salad with a fork. That way, I can enjoy another carb choice, like low-fat microwave popcorn, for a mid-afternoon snack. That's the great thing about this plan: You choose what's right for you on any given day.

✔ 1 small bunch of seedless grapes

✔ Chicken-Vegetable Salad (see the recipe following)

✔ 6 saltine crackers (1 carb choice)

✔ Cherry tomatoes

✔ Diet soda or a bottle of sparkling water

Chicken-Vegetable Salad

This chicken is delicious by itself or can be used on salads, in soups, or in other recipes. Paired with fresh fruits and veggies, it makes a great kid-friendly meal. And there are no hidden sugars or marinades that you find in the precooked, grilled chicken in the freezer section of your grocery store.

Preparation time: *10 minutes (plus at least 2 hours chilling time)*

Cooking time: *None*

Yield: *4 servings*

2 tablespoons lemon juice	*1 cup thinly sliced celery*
¼ cup reduced-fat Miracle Whip	*½ cup frozen green peas, thawed*
1 tablespoon minced parsley or parsley flakes	*5-ounce can (½ cup) sliced mushrooms, drained*
¼ teaspoon salt	*Paprika (optional)*
3 cups cooked chicken, cubed	*Pimento (optional)*

1 In a medium mixing bowl, combine lemon juice, mayonnaise, parsley, and salt. Add the chicken and the celery. Mix well.

2 Gently fold in the peas and mushrooms. Chill before serving. Garnish with pimento or paprika.

Note: *The small amount of green peas per serving is negligible for your carb count.*

Per serving: *Calories 238 (From Fat 91); Fat 10g (Saturated 2g); Cholesterol 83mg; Sodium 485mg; Carbohydrate 8g (Dietary Fiber 2g); Protein 28g.*

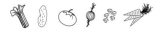

To take a salad for lunch, place the salad in a large resealable plastic bag with the dressing sealed in a separate sandwich-sized bag. Place the small bag in the larger one. At lunchtime, pour the dressing over the salad in the larger bag, seal tightly, and shake. No soggy salad, no messy cleanup, and no containers to tote back and forth between home and work. Assemble it the night before for even greater efficiency!

Satisfying Suppers

Unless your family has the luxury of similar departing times in the morning, dinner is probably the only meal at which every member is present and accounted for. Dinner deserves careful planning to ensure the right foods, but also to ensure pleasure and enjoyment. It's worth the extra effort because healthful food and pleasant feelings create a warm family atmosphere.

Evening nourishment

This is the winding down of your day and not the time to fuel up as breakfast and lunch are. Here you should be catching up on lean meats and green veggies. Keep your carb choices low at this time of day because you won't be burning them. Concentrate on building your meals around lean protein, fruit, and veggies.

Evening nourishment #1

This is a great way to enjoy a delicious variety of foods, with fairly easy preparation.

- ✔ Broiled Cinnamon Peaches (see Chapter 12 for recipe)
- ✔ Grilled chicken breast with teriyaki sauce
- ✔ Wild rice with mushrooms
- ✔ Steamed broccoli
- ✔ Pineapple Sundaes (see Chapter 11 for recipe)

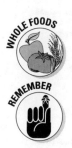

Count ½ cup wild rice as one carb choice. And count your pineapple sundae as one milk serving for the day because each sundae has ½ cup of light ice cream.

You can enjoy two to three servings of milk each day. For more information about dairy foods and low-carb dieting, take a peek at Chapter 7.

Evening nourishment #2

Roll up the leftover roast in butter lettuce leaves for a quick Green Light lunch the day after.

- ✔ Tossed green salad with cherry or grape tomatoes and red onion
- ✔ Reduced-fat salad dressing
- ✔ Betty's Busy Day Roast (see Chapter 12 for recipe)
- ✔ Corn Medley (see recipe following)
- ✔ Green Beans with Onions (see Chapter 12 for recipe)
- ✔ Iced tea with lemon wedges
- ✔ Thumbprint Cookies (see Chapter 11 for recipe)

Count ½ cup corn medley as one carb choice and two Thumbprint Cookies as one carb choice.

Evening nourishment #3

This is a great way to start working seafood into your diet if you're not a fan of it. If you're running low on carbohydrate choices for the day, skip the French bread and add another Green Light food.

- ✔ Baked Catfish Delight (see Chapter 12 for recipe)
- ✔ Zucchini-Tomato Bake (see Chapter 12 for recipe)
- ✔ Sliced French bread with garlic butter
- ✔ Peach Salad Cups (see Chapter 12 for recipe)
- ✔ Chocolate-Almond Crisps (see Chapter 12 for recipe)

Count each ½-inch slice of bread as one carb choice and three Chocolate-Almond Crisps as one carb choice. Indulge in each as your daily food plan permits.

Corn Medley

In this recipe, frozen corn is much better than its canned cousin. I find the frozen variety crisper, fresher, and even a bit sweeter. Very good!

Preparation time: *10 minutes*

Cooking time: *5 to 7 minutes*

Yield: *6 servings (1 serving equals one carbohydrate choice)*

10-ounce package frozen whole kernel corn	⅓ cup water	Salt and pepper to taste
½ cup chopped celery	2-ounce can sliced mushrooms, drained	Splash of balsamic vinegar (optional)
1 teaspoon powdered chicken bouillon	1 or 2 medium Roma tomatoes, diced	

1 In a saucepan, combine the corn, celery, bouillon, and ⅓ cup water. Bring to a boil. Cover and simmer until vegetables are tender, about 5 to 7 minutes.

2 Stir in the mushrooms and diced tomatoes; heat through. Season to taste with salt and pepper. Add a splash or two of balsamic vinegar, if desired.

Per serving: Calories 48 (From Fat 4); Fat 0g (Saturated 0g); Cholesterol 0mg; Sodium 190mg; Carbohydrate 11g (Dietary Fiber 2g); Protein 2g.

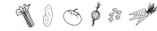

Company's coming

Don't think your food-related social life is over just because you're low-carb dieting. Invite people to your place so you can control the menu. Your guests will love these dishes and might not even notice that they're low in carbs.

Company's coming #1

This is a great menu if you're looking for a change from the everyday surf and turf, starting with the mushroom cocktail instead of shrimp cocktail. The most common version of Wellington is Beef Wellington, typically made with beef tenderloin stuffed with mushroom duxelle (minced mushrooms sautéed in butter and garlic) then wrapped in puff pastry or phyllo dough. This version is rich and delicious in its own right. Bon appetit!

- ✔ Mushroom Cocktail (see Chapter 11 for recipe)
- ✔ Bertie Jo's Salmon Wellington (see Chapter 12 for recipe)
- ✔ Savory Carrots (see Chapter 12 for recipe)
- ✔ Microwave Zucchini (see Chapter 12 for recipe)
- ✔ Peach-Yogurt Freeze (see Chapter 11 for recipe)
- ✔ Iced tea

Remember to count one carb for the puff pastry in Bertie Jo's Salmon Wellington.

Company's coming #2

This menu is a tasty one for breezy summer nights. The Key lime pudding cakes are tart and refreshing, and you make them in the microwave.

- ✔ Avocado-Orange Salad (see Chapter 12 for recipe)
- ✔ Cajun Shrimp (see Chapter 12 for recipe)
- ✔ Baked-Stuffed Potatoes (see recipe following)
- ✔ Harold's Stir-Fry (see Chapter 12 for recipe)
- ✔ Key Lime Pudding Cakes (see Chapter 11 for recipe)
- ✔ Ice tea or lemonade

Count one serving of Key Lime Pudding Cakes as ½ carb choice. You may want to double the portion size to one carb choice, for ease of counting — and because it's just plain good! Each serving of Baked Stuffed Potatoes is one carb choice.

☺ Baked Stuffed Potatoes

Preparation time: *1 hour, 10 minutes*

Cooking time: *20 minutes*

Yield: *6 servings (**1 serving equals one carbohydrate choice**)*

3 medium baking potatoes	*Dash pepper*
⅓ cup skim milk	*Dash paprika*
½ teaspoon salt	*Reduced-fat sharp cheddar cheese, grated*

1 Scrub potatoes; puncture skin with fork. Bake at 425 degrees for 1 hour. Cut potatoes in half lengthwise. Scoop out inside; mash.

2 Add milk, salt, and pepper to potato mash. Beat till fluffy, adding additional skim milk if needed. Pile lightly into shells; sprinkle with grated cheese. Return to oven until hot, about 10 minutes. Sprinkle with paprika.

Per serving: Calories 111 (From Fat 15); Fat 2g (Saturated 1g); Cholesterol 5mg; Sodium 268mg; Carbohydrate 20g (Dietary Fiber 2g); Protein 5g.

Snacking the Good-Carb Way

Wholesome snacks, chosen from nutritious foods, give a necessary lift. Also, when strategically placed in your day, they allow for good appetite control. Snacking can be a healthy part of your life. In fact, it's not at all unnatural to want to eat between meals. If you don't eat something about every four hours, your blood sugar dips, which can make you feel tired, cranky, and mentally sluggish.

Although many people believe that snacking causes weight gain, the reverse is often true. People who force themselves to resist snacks are more likely to be ravenous at mealtime and will probably overeat. Of course, the key to that is what you choose to snack on. Instead of pigging out on chips, approach snacking as you would any other meal. Be selective about what you eat and watch your portions of everything except for the Green Light foods. (For a list of the Green Light foods, check out Chapter 5.) Think of those between-meal bites as a chance to add vital nutrients to your diet and an opportunity to keep excess hunger in check.

Here are a few tips to get you going:

- ✔ **Develop a taste for fresh fruit and crunchy vegetables.**

- ✔ **For a satisfying snack, make a smoothie with low-fat yogurt, skim milk, and a soft fruit like strawberries, cantaloupe, or banana.** Remember to count the banana as a carb choice.

- ✔ **Use any of the appetizer and snack recipes in Chapter 11 or the Orange-Pineapple Delight recipe in Chapter 5.**

- ✔ **Buy resealable plastic bags.** The snack-size ones are great for more carb-intense choices. For easy snacking, you can make pre-portioned servings of Homemade Granola (see Chapter 12). You can make your own trail mix with peanuts, raisins, dried apricots, or whatever appeals to you and portion them out so they're easy to grab. It's great to keep the quart- or sandwich-size bags on hand for portioning out prepped Green Light veggies, like broccoli, pepper strips, and carrot sticks. These are quick snacks and easy salad fixings.

I often choose toothpicks as my snack-delivery system. Here are some of my favorite choices for snack kabobs:

- ✔ Pineapple chunks with a cube of ham

- ✔ Cooked chicken cubes with cucumber twists

- ✔ Roast beef cubes with chunks of dill pickle

- ✔ Cheese and ham cubes

- ✔ Luncheon meat cubes with cherry tomatoes

- ✔ Low-fat frankfurter bits dipped in mustard

Use Green Light foods stuffed with Green Light snacks to create edible bowls. They're pretty, filling, and you can eat the bowl when you're done!

- ✔ Tomato shell stuffed with cottage cheese

- ✔ Tomato shell stuffed with tuna salad

- ✔ Bell pepper shell with fillers

- ✔ Roll-ups:

    - Spread a slice of lunch meat with cream cheese or pimento cheese. Sprinkle with chopped pecans. Roll and secure with toothpick.

    - Stuff celery with egg salad, pimento cheese, cream cheese, or peanut butter.

Chapter 11

Savory Beginnings and Sweet Endings: Choosing the Best Recipes

*I*f you commit to this plan, do you have to toss out everything in your recipe box and pantry? Absolutely not. Review your family favorites and look for ways to incorporate them into your eating plan. You may be able to switch some of the carbo-hydrate choices to the fruits and vegetables that are free on this low-carb plan. Or you may be able to substitute a non-sugar sweetener, or use some unsaturated fats in place of saturated fats to bring a recipe into the plan. You may want to start forget-ting the meat-and-potatoes meal in favor of meat and salad with a touch of Yellow Light carbs. Whatever solutions you find, the healthy benefits will certainly be worth it. With a little practice, you won't even feel like you're dieting.

Checking Out Your Old Favorites

Tried-and-true recipes can become new again — and low-carb-friendly — if you know what to look for. Focus on giving food flavor without adding carbs and empty calories.

Try these simple changes to get started:

- ✔ Enjoy crunchy vegetables like jicama with your favorite salad instead of processed, store-bought crackers.

- ✔ Try making your favorite cheesecake recipe with Splenda rather than the normal white sugar.

- ✔ Substitute spaghetti squash for pasta.

- ✔ Cook fresh green beans in chicken broth instead of adding bacon.

- ✔ Substitute lower-fat healthy versions of canned cream soups in casseroles.

- ✔ Add nuts to salads instead of loading them up with full-fat dressing.

Assessing key recipe ingredients

The Whole Foods Eating Plan is not like some low-carb plans that require you to count every, single gram of carbohydrates. On the Whole Foods Eating Plan, lots of foods — like fruits (except bananas), leafy vegetables, lean meats, and cheese — don't count toward your daily carb tally at all. You just need to count the Yellow Light foods (starchy carbs, dairy foods, and good fats) and avoid the Red Light foods (which means don't yield to the temptation to indulge in excess Yellow Light foods).

When evaluating a recipe for its suitability on the Whole Foods Eating Plan, keep these tips in mind:

- ✔ **Fill up on the free Green Light fruits, veggies, and lean proteins.** Your hunger will be satisfied and your taste buds will be happy. *Remember:* I don't want you to be hungry, so enjoy Green Light foods as often as you like. Check out Chapter 5 for the lowdown.

- ✔ **Exercise caution and control with breads, cereals, legumes, pasta, refined-carb snacks, and other Yellow Light foods.** Remember not to exceed 5 carbohydrate choices, 2 cups of low-fat dairy, and 6 to 8 servings of good fats per day. Spend your carb choices wisely to get the most bang for your buck. For details on making your Yellow Light food choices, choosing your dairy servings, and understanding the truth about fats, take a peek at Chapters 6, 7, and 8, respectively.

- ✔ **Stop when you're about to exceed the amounts allowed in the Yellow Light section.** *Remember:* No food is *always* in the Red Light section. You only hit a Red Light when you exceed the limit.

Putting foods in their proper categories takes a little time. You may need to refer back to the concepts in Part III until you get the hang of it. Don't worry — you'll be a pro in no time.

Calculating your carb choices

Many recipes have a nutrition analysis that gives the total carbohydrate per serving. But this carbohydrate number includes all the carbohydrate in the recipe. Some of the carbohydrate in that recipe may be from fruits and veggies — and those are Green Light carbs for you.

In calculating the carb amount in a recipe on the Whole Foods Eating Plan, only count the carbohydrate provided by the *starchy* carbs. For example, the first recipe under "Appetizers and snacks," later in this chapter, is Marinated Mushrooms. All the ingredients in the recipe are Green Light foods except for a small amount of oil from the dressing. This recipe is considered a Green Light food, so enjoy! The Tasty Chicken Roll-Ups recipe calls for flour tortillas. One flour tortilla is a carbohydrate choice, and one flour tortilla makes seven roll-ups; therefore, seven roll-ups count as one carbohydrate choice.

You may need to review the information in Chapter 6 on controlling your carbohydrate intake. However, to help you get started, I have marked in **bold** the ingredients in the following recipes that contribute to your carbohydrate choices.

Adding Some New Recipes to Your Collection

If you'd rather get started without giving your old recipes a low-carb makeover, fear not. Here, I give you simple, delicious recipes that will help you succeed with your commitment to low-carb dieting. In this section, I cover healthy appetizers, snacks, beverages, and, believe it or not, desserts.

No foods (not even desserts) are absolutely off-limits on this dieting plan. If you watch your portion sizes and try the helpful tips that limit unnecessary sugars, you can still enjoy sweet treats and tasty snacks.

Appetizers and snacks

Appetizers are often the bane of healthy eating. Making frequent appearances on cocktail-party buffets, appetizers are often rich in fat or combined with an oil or butter base to buffer the impact of alcohol on the system. If guests fill up on these fat-laden goodies, they have no room to enjoy the main courses.

These easy appetizer recipes are light and healthy. They'll work for you and not against you in your quest for good health. Appetizers and snacks made from fruits and veggies can add up to an adequate amount of fiber before the main course is ever served.

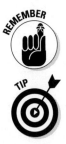

You don't always have to eat appetizers right before a meal. They're easy to make ahead and keep for yourself. Use them as a mid-afternoon or bedtime snack, or as something to grab when you have the munchies. Eat the Green Light ones freely.

If you're in a time crunch and need the mushrooms to marinate fast, you can try these quick marinating tips:

- ✔ **Quarter the mushrooms.** You create more surface area on the porous mushrooms to soak up the marinade fast. The chunky quarters should be big enough for your guests to spear.

- ✔ **Steam the mushrooms briefly in the microwave.** Place the mushrooms in a microwave-safe bowl. Cover with plastic wrap. Cut a few vent holes in the plastic, then microwave on high for 2 minutes. Allow the mushrooms to stand in the microwave for 3 minutes, then prepare as directed in the recipe.

🍅 Marinated Mushrooms

These mushrooms are great as a party appetizer, speared on colorful toothpicks. But they're so delicious you can serve them as the main ingredient in a hearty salad. They're complete in their own dressing!

Preparation time: *10 minutes (plus at least 1 hour marinating time)*

Cooking time: *None*

Yield: *2 cups*

1 pound small white button-type mushrooms, cleaned	*2 tablespoons chopped fresh parsley*
⅓ cup bottled vinaigrette dressing	*¼ teaspoon crushed red pepper*

1 Combine all ingredients in a non-metallic bowl.

2 Marinate at least 1 hour, preferably overnight in the refrigerator.

3 Spear onto colorful toothpicks and arrange on a platter.

Per ¼ cup serving: *Calories 35 (From Fat 17); Fat 2g (Saturated 0g); Cholesterol 0mg; Sodium 85mg; Carbohydrate 4g (Dietary Fiber 1g); Protein 2g.*

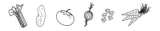

⟜ Fruit and Brie Kabobs

This is a great way to introduce kids to brie cheese. The sweet honey and crunchy almonds are irresistible. Adults love them, too. The flavor is so fresh and light, guests won't wonder where the crackers are.

Preparation time: *20 minutes*

Cooking time: *None*

Yield: *30 appetizers*

*One 3-pound cored, fresh pineapple
(or pineapple chunks, canned in own juice)*

*8 ounces round brie cheese, cut into
¾-inch cubes*

4 cups fresh strawberries

Leaf lettuce

2 tablespoons honey

1 tablespoon lemon juice

*1 tablespoon plus 1½ teaspoons chopped
almonds, toasted*

1 Cut the pineapple into 1-inch pieces or drain the canned pineapple chunks.

2 Thread the cheese cubes, pineapple, and strawberries onto 30 6-inch bamboo skewers.

3 Line a serving platter with the leaf lettuce. Arrange the kabobs over the lettuce.

4 Combine the honey and lemon juice; drizzle over the fruit kabobs. Sprinkle with the almonds.

Tip: *Check with the produce manager at your market to see if they can core a fresh pineapple for you. They usually have a handy machine that peels and cores this tasty fruit in one easy step, saving you some prep time.*

Per serving: *Calories 50 (From Fat 22); Fat 3g (Saturated 1g); Cholesterol 8mg; Sodium 48mg; Carbohydrate 6g (Dietary Fiber 1g); Protein 2g.*

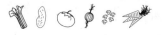

✏ *Apple-Cheese Spread*

If you're a dip fan, this is one recipe you have to try. The shredded apple gives a light crunch and incredible sweetness. Try different varieties of apples, like Fuji, Braeburn, and Granny Smith, for delicious variations.

Preparation time: *10 minutes (plus 4 hours chilling time)*

Cooking time: *None*

Yield: *1⅓ cups*

½ cup low-fat cottage cheese	*½ cup finely shredded reduced-fat cheddar cheese*	*½ cup shredded apple*
4 ounces (½ of an 8-ounce package) Neufchatel cheese, softened	*1 tablespoon brandy, optional*	*1 tablespoon finely chopped almonds, toasted*

1 Place the cottage cheese and Neufchatel cheese in a blender; process until smooth. Spoon into a small bowl. Add the remaining ingredients (except the almonds) to the cottage cheese and stir well. Top with the chopped almonds.

2 Cover and chill thoroughly, at least 4 hours.

Note: *Serve with apple or pear wedges, veggies slices, or melba toast rounds. (Just remember that melba toast rounds count as a carbohydrate — 9 rounds equals 1 carb choice.)*

Per 1 tablespoon serving: *Calories 25 (From Fat 15); Fat 2g (Saturated 1g); Cholesterol 5mg; Sodium 32mg; Carbohydrate 1g (Dietary Fiber 0g); Protein 2g.*

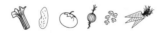

Zucchini-Shrimp Canapés

 Using zucchini slices in place of the bread rounds or crackers found in traditional canapés makes this elegant appetizer a Green Light food. Enjoy and feel a little pampered.

Preparation time: *20 minutes (plus 4 hours chilling time)*

Cooking time: *None*

Yield: *2 dozen*

4 ounces (½ of an 8-ounce package) Neufchatel cheese, softened	*¼ cup yellow or white onion, minced*	*4½-ounce can tiny shrimp, rinsed and drained*
½ cup reduced-calorie mayonnaise	*½ teaspoon dried dill*	*Fresh dill sprigs (optional)*
	2 large zucchini, cut crosswise into 24 ⅛-inch-thick slices	

1 Combine the first four ingredients in a small bowl; mix well. Cover and chill thoroughly, at least 4 hours.

2 Arrange the zucchini slices on a serving platter. Top each slice with 1 teaspoon of the chilled mixture. Top each canapé with 1 shrimp.

3 Garnish with dill sprigs, if desired.

Vary It! Toss the shrimp in a little lemon juice and pepper for a zesty variation.

Per serving: Calories 40 (From Fat 26); Fat 3g (Saturated 1g); Cholesterol 15mg; Sodium 69mg; Carbohydrate 2g (Dietary Fiber 0g); Protein 2g.

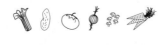

⟳ Jicama Chips

Jicama (see Figure 11-1) is a root vegetable that resembles a cross between a turnip and a potato. It has a fresh, slightly sweet flavor and a crisp texture similar to an apple or water chestnut. It's delicious raw or cooked. Keep a batch of these easy chips on hand for a satisfying snack anytime.

Preparation time: *10 minutes*

Cooking time: *None*

Yield: *4 servings, 8 chips each*

1 jicama, peeled and cut into ¼-inch slices

Cut jicama slices with assorted 1-inch cookie cutters. Store in an airtight container in the refrigerator.

Vary It! If you'd like a bit more flavor, try sprinkling these chips with lime juice and a touch of chili powder.

Per serving: Calories 40 (From Fat 0); Fat 0g (Saturated 0g); Cholesterol 0mg; Sodium 4mg; Carbohydrate 9g (Dietary Fiber 5g); Protein 1g.

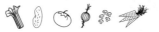

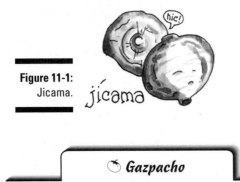

Figure 11-1:
Jicama.

🍅 Gazpacho

This chilled soup is a staple of the Spanish diet and it can be part of your low-carb eating plan, as well. The best thing about this soup is that you don't ever have to cook it, you can make it ahead of time, and you can eat as much as you want. It's made from Green Light, free foods.

Preparation time: *20 minutes (plus 8 hours chilling time)*

Cooking time: *None*

Yield: *6 cups*

3 medium tomatoes, peeled, seeded, and diced	1 medium cucumber, peeled and chopped
3 cups tomato juice	3 cloves garlic, minced
¼ cup diced onion	2 tablespoons chopped fresh parsley
¼ cup diced celery	1 teaspoon chopped fresh cilantro
1 medium-size green pepper, seeded and diced	3 tablespoons red wine vinegar
¼ cup sliced green onions	Dash of hot sauce
	⅛ teaspoon freshly ground pepper

1 Combine all ingredients in a large non-metallic bowl. Stir well.

2 Cover and chill at least 8 hours or overnight.

3 Stir well and ladle into soup bowls. Garnish with additional ground pepper and chopped fresh parsley or cilantro, if desired. Store in refrigerator for four or five days.

Tip: *Make sure you leave plenty of time for the flavors of this soup to meld or come together. The longer the soup sits, the more flavorful it becomes.*

Per 1 cup serving: Calories 61 (From Fat 3); Fat 0g (Saturated 0g); Cholesterol 0mg; Sodium 445mg; Carbohydrate 13g (Dietary Fiber 3g); Protein 3g.

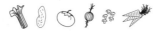

☽ *Bell-Pepper Nachos*

Bell peppers never had it so good! With this flavorful bean mixture, you won't even miss the tortilla chips.

Preparation time: *30 minutes*

Cooking time: *8 to 10 minutes*

Yield: *8 servings, 4 pieces per serving* **(1 carbohydrate choice)**

Nonstick vegetable cooking spray

1 medium green bell pepper

1 medium yellow or red bell pepper

2 roma tomatoes, seeded and chopped

¼ cup finely chopped onion

2 teaspoons chili powder

16-ounce can fat-free refried beans

½ cup shredded reduced-fat Monterey Jack cheese

2 tablespoons chopped fresh cilantro

¼ teaspoon hot pepper sauce

½ cup shredded reduced-fat sharp cheddar cheese

1 Preheat oven to 400 degrees. Spray large nonstick baking sheet with nonstick cooking spray; set aside.

2 Cut bell peppers in half; seed. Cut peppers into 2-x-1½-inch strips; cut strips into bite-sized triangles. Set aside.

3 Spray nonstick skillet with nonstick cooking spray. Add tomatoes, onion, and chili powder. Cook over medium heat 3 minutes or until onion is tender, stirring occasionally. Remove from the heat. Stir in refried beans, Monterey Jack cheese, cilantro, and pepper sauce.

4 Assemble the nachos. Top each pepper triangle with approximately 2 tablespoons of the bean mixture; sprinkle with cheddar cheese. Place the nachos on prepared baking sheets; cover with plastic wrap. Refrigerate up to 8 hours before serving. When ready to serve, remove the plastic wrap. Bake for 8 to 10 minutes, or until the cheese melts and the bean mixture is warmed through.

Vary It! *Mix it up a little and try different colored sweet peppers. Create a nacho rainbow: Add orange and purple sweet peppers.*

Per serving: *Calories 101 (From Fat 29); Fat 3g (Saturated 2g); Cholesterol 10mg; Sodium 292mg; Carbohydrate 12g (Dietary Fiber 4g); Protein 7g.*

Spicy Meatballs

A rimmed baking sheet helps you keep control of these tiny, round, tasty treats. As you pull out the tray to turn them, you'll see them roll around the cookie sheet a bit and will quickly appreciate the edge that saves them from the firey depths of your oven. Also, consider lining your baking sheet with foil to avoid messy cleanup later. And the amount of sugar in each meatball is negligible, so enjoy.

Preparation time: *10 minutes*

Cooking time: *12 to 15 minutes*

Yield: *60 meatballs*

1 pound extra-lean ground beef	*1 teaspoon salt*
1 tablespoon sugar or sugar-substitute equivalent	*½ cup chopped raisins*
¼ teaspoon ground cloves	*4-ounce can diced green chilies*
¼ teaspoon cinnamon	*1 egg, beaten*
	1 tablespoon dry sherry

1 Preheat oven to 500 degrees.

2 Combine all ingredients. Shape into tiny balls. Arrange balls on ungreased, rimmed baking sheet.

3 Bake for 12 to 15 minutes, turning occasionally. Serve with wooden picks.

Per serving: *Calories 17 (From Fat 5); Fat 1g (Saturated 0g); Cholesterol 5mg; Sodium 7mg; Carbohydrate 2g (Dietary Fiber 0g); Protein 1g.*

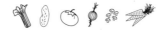

Artichoke-Ham Bites

This recipe is so easy and makes an elegant, sizzling snack. These are great appetizers for that spur-of-the-moment party or card game. Or you can just make them up for a filling snack.

Preparation time: *10 minutes (plus marinating time)*

Cooking time: *10 minutes*

Yield: *24 appetizers*

14-ounce can artichoke hearts	*⅛ teaspoon garlic powder*
½ cup low-calorie Italian salad dressing	*6 slices boiled ham*

1 Preheat oven to 300 degrees.

2 Drain artichoke hearts; cut in half. Combine the dressing and garlic powder; add the artichokes. Marinate several hours, or overnight; drain.

3 Cut the ham into 1-x-4-inch strips. Wrap one strip around each artichoke-heart half. Secure with a wooden toothpick.

Per serving: Calories 19 (From Fat 11); Fat 1g (Saturated 0g); Cholesterol 2mg; Sodium 126mg; Carbohydrate 2g (Dietary Fiber 0g); Protein 1g.

☞ *Mushroom Cocktail*

Move over shrimp cocktail! This mushroom cocktail is a delicious twist on the old favorite.

Preparation time: 10 minutes (plus chilling time)

Cooking time: None

Yield: 6 servings

⅓ cup ketchup	Lettuce leaves
1 tablespoon vinegar	1½ cups lettuce, shredded
¼ teaspoon prepared horseradish	12 fresh medium mushrooms, sliced

1 In a small bowl, blend the ketchup, vinegar, and horseradish. Chill for at least 1 hour. Line 6 sherbet cups with lettuce leaves; layer with shredded lettuce.

2 Arrange about ¼ cup sliced mushrooms atop each. Chill at least 30 minutes. Just before serving, drizzle each with 1 tablespoon of the ketchup mixture.

Per serving: Calories 25 (From Fat 2); Fat 0g (Saturated 0g); Cholesterol 0mg; Sodium 164mg; Carbohydrate 6g (Dietary Fiber 1g); Protein 1g.

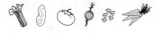

✆ Sharon's Zesty Cottage Cheese

This recipe makes a great filling snack. Feel free to substitute whatever veggies you have on hand for a quick snack with no shopping. Any blend of spices that you like works well. Cottage cheese is a great base to make just about any mix of veggie and seasonings. Experiment away!

Preparation time: *10 minutes*

Cooking time: *None*

Yield: *6 servings*

24-ounce container cottage cheese

2 roma tomatoes, seeded and diced

6 medium green onions, thinly sliced

1 medium cucumber, peeled, seeded, and diced

1 teaspoon seasoning salt

1 In a small mixing bowl, combine the cottage cheese, tomatoes, onion, cucumber, and seasoning salt; mix well.

2 Arrange ½ cup cottage cheese on the lettuce leaves for individual salads, if desired.

Per serving: *Calories 130 (From Fat 48); Fat 5g (Saturated 3g); Cholesterol 17mg; Sodium 617mg; Carbohydrate 6g (Dietary Fiber 1g); Protein 15g.*

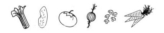

Tasty Chicken Roll-Ups

Try these roll-ups as an appetizer for a group, or keep the uncut roll-ups handy in the fridge for a quick snack. These also make a delicious quick lunch for kids.

Preparation time: *10 minutes (plus 2 hours chilling time)*

Cooking time: *None*

Yield: *35 roll-ups, 7 roll-ups per serving* **(1 carbohydrate choice per serving)**

¼ cup light cream cheese, softened

3 tablespoons canned chopped green chilies

2 teaspoons tomato sauce

½ teaspoon chili powder

Five 7-inch flour tortillas

Two 2½-ounce packages very thinly sliced chicken

2 tablespoons chopped ripe olives

1 Beat cream cheese in a bowl at medium speed with an electric mixer until smooth. Add chilies, tomato sauce, and chili powder; stir well. Spread over tortillas.

2 Top with chicken and olives. Roll up the tortillas jellyroll fashion, as shown in Figure 11-2. Cover with plastic wrap; chill 2 hours. Cut into 1-inch pieces.

Per serving: Calories 171 (From Fat 46); Fat 5g (Saturated 2g); Cholesterol 33mg; Sodium 173mg; Carbohydrate 17g (Dietary Fiber 1g); Protein 14g.

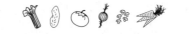

ROLLING UP A TORTILLA FOR ROLL-UPS

Figure 11-2:
Rolling up
tortillas
jellyroll-
style.

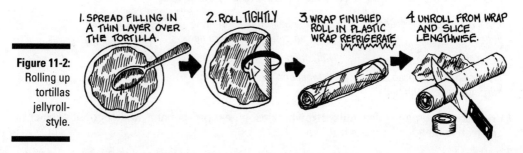

1. SPREAD FILLING IN A THIN LAYER OVER THE TORTILLA.

2. ROLL TIGHTLY

3. WRAP FINISHED ROLL IN PLASTIC WRAP REFRIGERATE

4. UNROLL FROM WRAP AND SLICE LENGTHWISE.

Beverages

These beverage recipes are great additions to any breakfast, lunch, or dinner. You'll welcome them with a good book, a roaring fire, and a rainy day. Enjoy these nourishing beverages any time.

☞ Four-Fruit Shake

This shake is a great combination of delicious fruits, but don't limit yourself to this recipe. Keep your proportions of fruit, yogurt, and liquid the same, but feel free to substitute any fruits you have on hand. Just remember to count the banana (if you're using one) in your carbohydrate count for the day. One of my favorite variations substitutes freshly peeled kiwi for half the strawberries. Mango and papaya are also great choices. Blueberries make an excellent addition as well, and kids love the funky color to spice up their breakfast routine.

Preparation time: *5 minutes*

Cooking time: *None*

Yield: *Six 1-cup servings (¼ carbohydrate choice per serving)*

1 cup unsweetened orange juice	8-ounce can unsweetened crushed pineapple, undrained	1 cup ice cubes
1 cup skim milk	1 medium-size ripe banana	Fresh strawberry slices, optional
1½ cups fresh or frozen strawberries, washed and hulled	¼ teaspoon coconut extract	

1 Combine the orange juice, milk, strawberries, pineapple, banana, and coconut extract in an electric blender; process until smooth.

2 Add the ice cubes, and process until smooth. Pour into glasses and garnish with strawberry slices, if desired. Serve immediately.

Vary It! *For an ultra-smooth shake, substitute crushed ice for ice cubes. Your blender will do less work and thank you for it.*

Per serving: *Calories 85 (From Fat 4); Fat 0g (Saturated 0g); Cholesterol 0mg; Sodium 23mg; Carbohydrate 19g (Dietary Fiber 2g); Protein 2g.*

☞ Peppermint Cocoa

This is a great fireside treat after a long day of shoveling driveways and building snowmen.

Preparation time: *3 minutes*

Cooking time: *5 to 7 minutes*

Yield: *Four ½-cup servings*

3 tablespoons unsweetened cocoa	⅛ teaspoons salt	2 cups skim milk
3 tablespoons Splenda	⅓ cup water	¼ teaspoon peppermint extract

1 In a large saucepan, combine the cocoa, Splenda, salt, and water; mix well.

2 Cook over medium heat, stirring constantly, until the mixture comes to a rolling boil. Gradually stir in the milk and peppermint. Heat just to boiling. Serve hot.

Tip: For a special holiday treat, look for sugar-free candy canes and use them to decorate and stir your cocoa at the same time.

Per serving: Calories 54 (From Fat 5); Fat 1g (Saturated 0g); Cholesterol 3mg; Sodium 137mg; Carbohydrate 9g (Dietary Fiber 1g); Protein 5g.

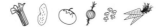

☕ Hot Tomato Refresher

GREEN LIGHT This warm beverage is ideal as a help-yourself appetizer, served in a slow cooker.

Preparation time: *5 minutes*

Cooking time: *8 to 10 minutes*

Yield: *Twelve 4-ounce servings*

Two 24-ounce cans vegetable juice cocktail	*½ teaspoon ground allspice*
2 tablespoons lemon juice	*Lemon slices (optional)*
2 teaspoons Worcestershire sauce	

1 In a large saucepan, combine all the ingredients, except the lemon slices. Heat through, but do not boil.

2 Just before serving, float thin lemon slices atop the hot beverage, if desired.

Vary It! You can add 1½ cups of vodka to create a warm wintry Bloody Mary. Just make sure you count one carb choice for each serving.

Per serving: Calories 25 (From Fat 0); Fat 0g (Saturated 0g); Cholesterol 0mg; Sodium 299mg; Carbohydrate 5g (Dietary Fiber 1g); Protein 1g.

Desserts

Desserts can be heavenly and are a highly anticipated ending to a meal. However, topping off an impressive meal with a disastrously rich dessert can leave you feeling stuffed and sluggish. Fresh fruit can be a far better conclusion for all your guests. Fruit in either cup, salad, or sherbet form can serve as a "lightener" during, as well as after, a meal. If you want a little richer post-meal treat, dessert may be a good place to spend one or two of those five carbohydrate choices you're allowed each day. But it's nice to know that with these great fruit dessert recipes, you don't have to!

Poached Pears with Raspberry-Almond Purée

GREEN LIGHT

This elegant dessert is a great finish for an intimate dinner with friends.

Preparation time: *20 minutes*

Cooking time: *40 to 50 minutes (plus cooling time)*

Yield: *4 servings*

1½ cups water	*4 whole pears, peeled, stems left on*
¾ cup Splenda	*10 ounces frozen raspberries, thawed*
½ teaspoon cinnamon	*¼ teaspoon almond extract*
Juice from 1 lemon, approximately 3 tablespoons	*Chopped almonds*

1 Bring water, Splenda, cinnamon, and lemon juice to a boil in a covered, deep saucepan. Add the pears to the boiling liquid. If the pears are not covered, add water until they are. Return to a simmer, cover, and cook 20 to 30 minutes or until firm-tender. Cool in cooking liquid, until cool enough to handle.

2 Gently core the pears from the bottom, removing the seeds. Puree the raspberries and almond extract in a blender.

3 Serve raspberry puree over or under the pears. Sprinkle with chopped almonds.

Per serving: Calories 165 (From Fat 19); Fat 2g (Saturated 0g); Cholesterol 0mg; Sodium 1mg; Carbohydrate 38g (Dietary Fiber 5g); Protein 2g.

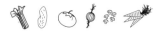

☞ *Peach Yogurt Freeze*

This is a great treat on a hot day, or anytime you need a frozen treat. Experiment with whatever fruits are your favorite. It's great with strawberries or raspberries if you don't mind a few seeds! And to speed up the preparation, look for frozen fruit with no added sugar. It can save you valuable peeling and coring time!

Preparation time: *40 minutes*

Cooking time: *5 minutes (plus freezing time)*

Yield: *Eight 1-cup servings* ***(each serving equals one serving of milk and free fruit)***

1 envelope unflavored gelatin (¼ ounce)

½ cup cold water

2 eggs

⅓ cup Splenda

½ cup unsweetened orange juice

Two 16-ounce cartons low-fat vanilla yogurt

3 cups peeled, chopped fresh peaches

1 Soften the gelatin in cold water in a small saucepan; let stand 1 minute. Cook over medium heat, stirring constantly, until gelatin dissolves. Set aside.

2 Beat the eggs and Splenda until thick and lemon colored. Stir in the reserved gelatin mixture, the orange juice, and the yogurt. Place the peaches in an electric blender or food processor; process until smooth. Add the pureed peaches to the yogurt mixture; stir well.

3 Pour the peach mixture into the freezer can of a hand-turned or electric ice-cream freezer. Freeze according to the manufacturer's instructions. Scoop the peach mixture into individual dessert bowls, and serve immediately.

Per serving: Calories 108 (From Fat 19); Fat 2g (Saturated 1g); Cholesterol 56mg; Sodium 55mg; Carbohydrate 18g (Dietary Fiber 1g); Protein 6g.

If you're a dessert freak, an ice-cream freezer is a great addition to your low-carb lifestyle. If you make your own yogurt, ice cream, or sorbet, you can control the amount of sugar you add to any recipe and ensure that you're using delicious fresh fruit every time. Most freezers come with a recipe book that includes sugar-free and low-sugar recipes.

☞ Maple Apple Rings

These apple rings are a great dessert, but they also make a great addition to any brunch. Vary the baking time based on your preference. The apples are crisp-tender after about 15 minutes, but if you like really tender apples, go for 30 minutes.

Preparation time: *25 minutes*

Cooking time: *15 minutes*

Yield: *4 servings*

4 medium baking apples, cored and thinly sliced into rings	3 tablespoons reduced-calorie maple syrup	½ teaspoon ground cinnamon
	1 tablespoon tub margarine, melted	⅛ teaspoon ground nutmeg
		¼ cup sliced almonds

1 Preheat oven to 350 degrees.

2 Arrange the apple rings evenly in a 1½-quart baking dish sprayed with nonstick cooking spray. Combine the syrup, margarine, cinnamon, and nutmeg, stirring well. Spoon the syrup mixture evenly over the apples. Sprinkle the almonds over the syrup mixture. Cover the dish. Bake 15 minutes or until apples are tender.

Per serving: *Calories 161 (From Fat 57); Fat 6g (Saturated 1g); Cholesterol 0mg; Sodium 60mg; Carbohydrate 27g (Dietary Fiber 5g); Protein 2g.*

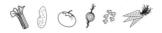

☞ Pineapple Sundaes

Pineapple is so naturally sweet, you don't need the heavy or even light syrup found in some canned fruit. Look for it canned in its own juice. If you have some extra fat choices for the day, consider adding some toasted nuts on top. Yummy!

Preparation time: *15 minutes*

Cooking time: *20 minutes*

Yield: *6 servings* **(each sundae equals one serving of milk and free fruit)**

8-ounce can pineapple tidbits in own juice	2 teaspoons cornstarch	⅛ teaspoon ground nutmeg
	3 tablespoons raisins	½ teaspoon vanilla extract
Brown sugar substitute equivalent to 2 tablespoons	2 teaspoons tub margarine	3 cups light vanilla ice cream
1 tablespoon water	¼ teaspoon ground cinnamon	1 tablespoon unsweetened flaked coconut, toasted

1 Drain the pineapple, reserving the juice. Set the pineapple aside. Combine the reserved juice, brown sugar substitute, water, and cornstarch in a small non-aluminum saucepan; stir well. Cook over medium heat until thickened, stirring constantly. Stir in the pineapple, raisins, margarine, cinnamon, and nutmeg. Cook over low heat, stirring frequently, until thoroughly heated. Stir in the vanilla.

2 To serve, place ½ cup light ice cream in individual dessert dishes. Spoon 3 tablespoons warm pineapple mixture over each serving of ice cream. Sprinkle ½ teaspoon coconut over each serving. Serve immediately.

Per serving: Calories 191 (From Fat 56); Fat 6g (Saturated 3g); Cholesterol 35mg; Sodium 62mg; Carbohydrate 32g (Dietary Fiber 1g); Protein 3g.

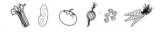

🍃 Sparkling Fresh Fruit Cup

This is a quick and elegant dessert. If any fruit in the recipe is not in season, feel free to substitute your favorites. You can even substitute canned fruit if absolutely necessary, but I recommend draining the fruit before combining it with the sparkling cider.

Preparation time: 25 minutes

Cooking time: None

Yield: 8 servings

4 medium-size fresh pears, cored and diced

2 tablespoons lemon juice

2 cups halved fresh strawberries

¾ pound fresh plums, pitted and thinly sliced

2 cups peeled, diced fresh peaches

2 cups sparkling apple cider, chilled

Fresh mint sprigs (optional)

1 Place diced pears in a large bowl, and sprinkle with lemon juice; toss gently. Add strawberries, plums, and peaches; toss gently to combine.

2 To serve, place 1 cup fruit mixture in individual dessert cups. Pour ¼ cup sparkling apple cider over each serving. Garnish with fresh mint sprigs, if desired. Serve immediately.

Per serving: Calories 138 (From Fat 8); Fat 1g (Saturated 0g); Cholesterol 0mg; Sodium 1mg; Carbohydrate 35g (Dietary Fiber 4g); Protein 1g.

Cranberry-Grape Sorbet

Sorbet is so easy to make but can really impress your guests. You can substitute diet grapefruit soda (like Fresca) or lemon-lime soda for the apple juice, if you prefer.

Preparation time: *15 minutes (plus freezing time)*

Cooking time: *None*

Yield: *Twelve ½-cup servings*

2½ cups cran-grape juice cocktail	1 egg white
½ cup sparkling apple juice	1 tablespoon Splenda

1 Pour the cran-grape juice cocktail into 2 freezer-safe trays; freeze until almost firm. Spoon the mixture into a large mixing bowl, and beat at high speed of an electric mixer until slushy. Gently stir in the sparkling apple juice. Using an electric mixer, beat the egg white (at room temperature) at high speed for 1 minute. Add the Splenda, beating until soft peaks form. Carefully fold the beaten egg white into the juice mixture.

2 Pour into the freezer can of a hand-turned or electric ice-cream freezer. Freeze according to the manufacturer's instructions. Scoop the sorbet into individual dessert bowls, and serve immediately.

Per serving: *Calories 36 (From Fat 1); Fat 0g (Saturated 0g); Cholesterol 0mg; Sodium 6mg; Carbohydrate 9g (Dietary Fiber 0g); Protein 0g.*

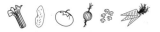

Frosty Fruit Cup

This is a great way to spruce up the age-old fruit cup. It's a great alternative to ice cream on a hot day — and it's a Green Light food. What more could you ask for?

Preparation time: *10 minutes (plus freezing time)*

Cooking time: *None*

Yield: *8 servings*

15-ounce can pineapple chunks, in own juice	Few drops green food coloring
16 ounces diet lemon-lime carbonated beverage	1 cup seedless green grapes
	2 cups cantaloupe balls
2 tablespoons lime juice	Mint sprigs, if desired

1 Drain the pineapple, reserving the juice. Combine the reserved juice, carbonated beverage, lime juice, and food coloring; stir. Pour into a 3-cup refrigerator-safe tray; freeze just to a mush, about 2 to 2½ hours. A few stirs every 30 minutes or so will help keep it slushy.

2 Combine the pineapple chunks, grapes, and cantaloupe. Break the frozen mixture apart with a fork, if necessary. Spoon into 8 sherbet glasses; top with fruits. Garnish with mint sprigs, if desired.

Per serving: Calories 61 (From Fat 2); Fat 0g (Saturated 0g); Cholesterol 0mg; Sodium 16mg; Carbohydrate 15g (Dietary Fiber 1g); Protein 1g.

☙ Chocolate-Almond Crisps

These tasty morsels are great for chocoholics everywhere. And you can't get a better source of vitamin E than almonds. Healthy chocolate "cookies" — who knew it was possible?

Preparation time: *15 minutes*

Cooking time: *40 minutes*

Yield: *12 dozen servings, 3 crisps per serving* **(1 carbohydrate choice per serving)**

2 egg whites at room temperature

¾ cup plus 2 tablespoons sifted powdered sugar

3 tablespoons plus 1½ teaspoons unsweetened cocoa

¼ cup semisweet chocolate mini-morsels

¼ cup finely chopped blanched almonds

½ teaspoon almond extract

Vegetable cooking spray

1 Preheat oven to 300 degrees.

2 Beat egg whites at high speed of electric mixer for 1 minute. Combine the sugar and cocoa; gradually add the sugar mixture to the egg whites, 1 tablespoon at a time, beating until stiff peaks form and the sugar dissolves, 2 to 4 minutes. Fold in mini-morsels, almonds, and almond extract.

3 Drop by teaspoonfuls, 1 inch apart, onto cookie sheets that have been lined with parchment paper. Bake for 40 minutes or until set. Cool slightly on cookie sheets; gently remove to wire racks, and cool completely. Store in an airtight container.

Per serving: Calories 7 (From Fat 2); Fat 0g (Saturated 0g); Cholesterol 0mg; Sodium 1mg; Carbohydrate 1g (Dietary Fiber 0g); Protein 0g.

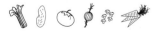

☞ *Peanutty Cupcakes*

These delicious cupcakes are a great treat for kids and adults. Kids of all ages race to the creamy peanut-butter filling.

Preparation time: *25 minutes*

Cooking time: *20 minutes*

Yield: *12 cupcakes (**1 carbohydrate choice per serving**)*

2 ounces Neufchatel cheese, softened	*1 egg*
3 tablespoons no-sugar-added creamy peanut butter	*½ teaspoon vanilla extract*
	¾ cup all-purpose flour
1 tablespoon honey	*½ teaspoon baking soda*
½ cup quick cooking oats, uncooked	*1 teaspoon ground cinnamon*
¾ cup boiling water	*½ teaspoon ground cloves*
⅓ cup vegetable oil	*¼ teaspoon ground nutmeg*
Brown sugar substitute equivalent to ½ cup packed brown sugar	*⅛ teaspoon salt*

1 Preheat oven to 375 degrees. Combine the Neufchatel cheese, peanut butter, and honey in a small bowl, stirring well; set aside. Combine the oats and boiling water in a small bowl, stirring well. Set aside, and let cool.

2 Gradually combine the oil and sugar, beating well at medium speed. Add the egg and vanilla, beating well. In a separate bowl, combine the flour, soda, cinnamon, cloves, nutmeg, and salt. Alternately add the flour mixture and oatmeal mixture to the creamed mixture, beginning and ending with the flour mixture. Mix well after each addition, scraping the sides of the bowl often.

3 Spoon ⅔ cup of batter into each of 12 paper-lined muffin cups. Put ½ tablespoon of the peanut butter mixture on top of the batter. Bake for 20 minutes. Remove the cupcakes from pans, and let cool on wire racks.

Per serving: *Calories 160 (From Fat 90); Fat 10g (Saturated 2g); Cholesterol 21mg; Sodium 116mg; Carbohydrate 19g (Dietary Fiber 1g); Protein 3g.*

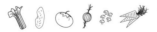

Reusable, nonstick baking sheets work great for lining cookie sheets. A product from France made by Silpat replaces pan-greasing or cooking spray. The Silpat sheet makes for easy cleanup. You can find them in most kitchen stores.

☜ Key Lime Pudding Cakes

These tasty desserts are pre-portioned so it's easy to stick to your eating plan.

Preparation time: 15 minutes

Cooking time: 5 minutes (plus 4 minutes standing time)

Yield: 6 servings (½ **carbohydrate choice per serving; if using sugar instead of Splenda, 1 carbohydrate choice per serving**)

¼ cup plus 2 tablespoons Splenda	2 tablespoons key lime juice
⅛ cup all-purpose flour	1 tablespoon lime zest
¼ teaspoon salt	Vegetable cooking spray
2 eggs, separated, at room temperature	Lime slices, fresh berries, fresh mint sprigs for garnish (optional)
¾ cup skim milk	

1 Combine the Splenda, flour, and salt in a medium bowl; set aside. Beat the egg yolks at the high speed of an electric mixer until thick and lemon colored; add the milk and lime juice, beating well. Mix in the dry ingredients; beat well. Set aside.

2 Beat the egg whites at the high speed of an electric mixer until soft peaks form. Gently fold the egg whites and lime zest into the milk–egg yolk mixture. Pour the batter evenly into six 6-ounce custard cups that have been coated with cooking spray.

3 Place 3 custard cups in the microwave. Microwave, uncovered, at medium-high (70-percent power) for 2 to 2½ minutes, rotating a half-turn after 1 minute. Let stand 2 minutes. Repeat with the remaining custard cups. If desired, garnish with berries, lime slices, and fresh mint sprigs. Serve warm.

Per serving: Calories 68 (From Fat 16); Fat 2g (Saturated 1g); Cholesterol 71mg; Sodium 134mg; Carbohydrate 9g (Dietary Fiber 0g); Protein 4g.

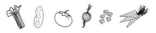

☃ Thumbprint Cookies

These cookies will quickly become holiday favorites. Try any flavor of all-fruit spread that appeals to you. Raspberry and apricot make delicious variations.

Preparation time: *30 minutes*

Cooking time: *8 to 9 minutes*

Yield: *10 servings, 2 cookies per serving* **(1 carbohydrate choice per serving)**

8-ounce package Sweet 'n Low sugar-free
low-fat yellow cake mix

3 tablespoons orange juice

2 teaspoons grated orange peel

½ teaspoon almond extract

4 teaspoons peach all-fruit spread

2 tablespoons almonds, chopped

1 Preheat oven to 350 degrees. Spray baking sheets with nonstick cooking spray.

2 Beat the cake mix, orange juice, orange peel, and almond extract in a medium bowl with an electric mixer at medium speed for 2 minutes, until the mixture looks crumbly. Increase the speed to medium and beat 2 minutes or until smooth dough forms. Dough will be very sticky. Coat your hands with nonstick cooking spray. Roll the dough into 1-inch balls.

3 Place the balls 2½ inches apart on prepared baking sheets. Press the center of each ball with your thumb. Fill each thumbprint with ¼ teaspoon fruit spread. Sprinkle with nuts. Bake 8 to 9 minutes or until cookies are light golden brown and lose their shininess. Do not over bake. Remove to wire racks; cool completely.

Per serving: Calories 87 (From Fat 44); Fat 5g (Saturated 1g); Cholesterol 0mg; Sodium 15mg; Carbohydrate 12g (Dietary Fiber 1g); Protein 1g.

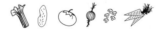

☼ *Cranberry Ice Delight*

Try this ending to your Thanksgiving dinner. It's more refreshing than pumpkin pie, with a lot less sugar and fat. I'll give thanks for that.

Preparation time: *5 minutes (plus freezing time)*

Cooking time: *8 minutes*

Yield: *6 servings*

½ cup Splenda	*2 cups reduced-calorie cranberry juice cocktail, divided*
½ envelope unflavored gelatin, approximately 1½ teaspoons	*1 tablespoon lemon juice*
Dash salt	

1 In a saucepan, combine the Splenda, gelatin, and salt. Stir in 1 cup of the cranberry juice cocktail. Heat and stir over medium heat until the Splenda and gelatin dissolve. Remove from the heat. Stir in the additional 1 cup of cranberry juice cocktail and 1 tablespoon lemon juice.

2 Freeze in a 3-cup refrigerator tray until firm. Break into chunks; in a chilled bowl, beat with an electric mixer until smooth. Return the cranberry mixture to the tray; freeze until firm. To serve, break into chunks with a fork and spoon into individual dessert dishes.

Remember: *Don't forget to chill the beater along with the mixing bowl, or you'll have a super-slushy mess on your hands.*

Per serving: *Calories 26 (From Fat 0); Fat 0g (Saturated 0g); Cholesterol 0mg; Sodium 27mg; Carbohydrate 6g (Dietary Fiber 0g); Protein 1g.*

Chapter 12

Entrees and Side Dishes

In This Chapter

▶ Getting your comfort-food fix the low-carb way

▶ Planning healthy entrees and side dishes from Green Light foods

▶ Keeping carbohydrates low in your total meal

*T*he heart and soul of any meal is the all-important main dish. In this chapter, you'll find easy recipes that treat your body right and satisfy your taste buds. I show you how to pair these main dishes with delicious side dishes, adding variety and interest to any table.

From comfort foods, to must-have snacks, you're sure to find something in this chapter to make even the pickiest eaters happy.

Comfort Foods

How could you live without comfort food? Comfort foods are the delicious foods of childhood; the foods you crave when you're worried, sick, or anxious; and the foods you prepare to show people how much you love them.

Even though many eating plans don't allow for comfort foods, the Whole Foods Eating Plan makes room for these delicious treats, making sure you don't have to give up the foods you love. Savory chicken and vegetables, tasty meatloaf, and hearty soups all make an appearance in the plan. Try your hand at converting your own family favorites to low-carb sensations by calculating the Yellow Light carbs. (For help on this, check out Chapter 11.) Let's face it, sometimes we can all use a little extra tender-loving care.

Main dish mainstays

These delicious main courses can be a meal in themselves, or you can pair them with a garden salad or another side dish for a hearty meal. Try combining a cup of Jim's Sausage Soup and Baked Chicken with Winter Vegetables for a delicious, satisfying, low-carb meal. Polish it off with the Sparkling Fresh Fruit Cup from Chapter 11 for a true treat. Experiment to find your favorite combinations.

Baked Chicken with Winter Vegetables

An oven browning bag makes this chicken crispy and the vegetables flavorful and tender. Typically, people use oven bags for cooking turkeys at holidays, but you can use them to cook meats and veggies any day of the year. Look for these handy bags in the grocery store near the foil, plastic wrap, and plastic bags.

Preparation time: *30 minutes*

Cooking time: *1 hour*

Yield: *8 servings (*¹/₈ **carbohydrate choice per serving)**

⅓ pound fresh or frozen Brussels sprouts, cleaned and stemmed

2 medium tomatoes, cut into wedges

⅓ pound carrots, peeled and cut into ¼-inch diagonal slices

1 acorn squash (about 8 ounces), peeled, seeded, and cubed

¼ cup chopped onion

1 teaspoon dried basil leaves

½ teaspoon dry mustard

¼ teaspoon salt

¼ teaspoon pepper

3½-pound broiler fryer chicken, cut up and skinned

1 large oven browning bag

1 Preheat oven to 350 degrees. Combine sprouts, tomatoes, carrots, squash, onion, basil, mustard, salt, and pepper in a large bowl; toss well. Set aside.

2 Trim the excess fat from the chicken. Rinse the chicken with cold water; pat dry. Place the chicken in an oven browning bag prepared according to the package instructions. Place the reserved vegetable mixture in a bag around the chicken. Seal the bag according to the package instructions, cutting slits in the top of the bag. Place the bag in a 13-x-9-x-2-inch baking dish; bake for 1 hour or until chicken and vegetables are tender.

Per serving: Calories 183 (From Fat 54); Fat 6g (Saturated 2g); Cholesterol 68mg; Sodium 156mg; Carbohydrate 9g (Dietary Fiber 3g); Protein 24g.

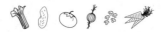

Brussels sprouts have a bad reputation with some people. But if you clean them properly, they can be an easy, delicious part of your regular diet. Remove their discolored leaves, cut off the stem ends, and wash them thoroughly. Cut a shallow X in the base of each sprout. This X allows the sprout to pick up the flavor of the cooking sauce or broth and become extremely tender. (Check out Figure 12-1 for instructions on preparing Brussels sprouts.)

PREPARING BRUSSELS SPROUTS

RINSE SPROUTS. REMOVE ANY SHRIVELED, OUTER LEAVES. TRIM WOODY BOTTOMS WITH A SHARP KNIFE AND INCISE AN 'X' ON THE BOTTOM.

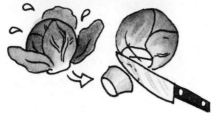

Figure 12-1: Preparing Brussels sprouts.

Betty's Busy-Day Roast

This recipe is delicious with just about any lean cut of meat. Try it with brisket, London broil, or anything you have in your freezer. Cheaper cuts of meat can become tender and juicy when cooked for long periods of time at low temperatures.

Preparation time: *10 minutes*

Cooking time: *8 hours*

Yield: *8 servings*

6-pound beef roast

2 teaspoons salt

2 teaspoons pepper

1 tablespoon garlic salt

¼ cup Worcestershire sauce

1 Preheat the oven to 225 degrees. Trim the excess fat from the roast. Cover with salt, pepper, and garlic salt.

2 Place the roast in a roasting pan, pour the Worcestershire sauce over it, and cover tightly. Bake for 8 hours. Skim the fat from the pan juices; reserve 1 cup of the juice to serve over the meat.

Tip: Make more roast than you'll need. The leftovers make great lettuce-wrap fillings and salad ingredients. Just slice it and place it on top of your favorite greens or chunk it up and serve it in butter lettuce cups. Delicious!

Per serving: Calories 510 (From Fat 222); Fat 25g (Saturated 11g); Cholesterol 163mg; Sodium 1,227mg; Carbohydrate 2g (Dietary Fiber 0g); Protein 66g.

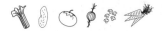

No-Fail Meatloaf

This meatloaf might become a part of your weekly rotation. Serve it with Savory Carrots or Summer Squash Medley, both later in this chapter, for an extra Green Light punch to your daily plan.

Preparation time: *15 minutes*

Cooking time: *1 to 1½ hours*

Yield: *8 servings (½ carbohydrate choice per serving)*

1½ pounds extra-lean ground beef	*¼ teaspoon pepper*
Three 8-ounce cans tomato sauce	**3 tablespoons brown sugar**
1 egg, beaten	*2 tablespoons prepared mustard*
1 cup dried bread crumbs	*2 tablespoons Worcestershire sauce*
1 tablespoon dried onion	*3 tablespoons vinegar*
1½ teaspoons salt	

1 Preheat oven to 350 degrees. Lightly mix the ground beef, 1 can of the tomato sauce, egg, bread crumbs, onion, salt, and pepper. Form a loaf from the mixture. Place in a shallow baking dish.

2 In a small bowl, combine the brown sugar, mustard, Worcestershire sauce, vinegar, and the remaining 2 cans of tomato sauce. Pour over the meatloaf and bake uncovered 1 to 1½ hours.

Tip: *To make this meatloaf a Green Light food, cut out the bread crumbs and use brown sugar substitute for the brown sugar.*

Per serving: *Calories 243 (From Fat 65); Fat 7g (Saturated 3g); Cholesterol 50mg; Sodium 1,171mg; Carbohydrate 26g (Dietary Fiber 1g); Protein 17g.*

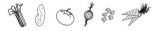

Bun-Less Bacon Cheeseburgers

Try these delicious bacon-cheeseburger-like tasties without a bun for a true treat. Serve with a green salad for a great summertime meal.

Preparation time: *10 minutes*

Cooking time: *10 minutes*

Yield: *6 servings*

1 pound extra-lean ground beef	*1½ tablespoons ketchup*
1 egg, beaten	*1½ tablespoons Worcestershire sauce*
½ cup reduced-fat sharp cheddar cheese, grated	*½ teaspoon salt*
	¼ teaspoon pepper
3 tablespoons onion, finely chopped	*6 slices turkey bacon or other lean bacon*

1 Mix well all ingredients except bacon. Form into 6 thick patties. Wrap bacon around each patty and secure with toothpicks.

2 Broil either under a broiler or on a grill until the bacon appears well done, approximately 10 minutes, turning once during cooking.

Per serving: Calories 179 (From Fat 97); Fat 11g (Saturated 4g); Cholesterol 75mg; Sodium 502mg; Carbohydrate 3g (Dietary Fiber 0g); Protein 17g.

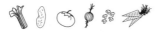

Hearty soups

Nothing spells comfort to your family more than a hearty soup. Spend a carbohydrate choice here and add a fruity dessert to complete the meal. If possible, start your soup at least a couple hours before serving. I often make my soups the night or day before and refrigerate them overnight. Any excess fat solidifies on top, for easy removal. For an added bonus, the soup thickens in the fridge, making it extra delicious the next day.

Navy Bean Soup

I often keep a batch of this soup in the freezer for quick weeknight meals. It's an easy one to double and save the leftovers. Twice the results for the same effort — that's my kind of meal.

Preparation time: *30 minutes (plus standing time overnight)*

Cooking time: *Approximately 2 hours*

Yield: *6 servings* (*2 carbohydrate choices per serving*)

1½ cups dried navy beans	4 cups water
Vegetable cooking spray	1 tablespoons plus 1 teaspoon chicken-flavored bouillon granules
1 medium onion, chopped	
½ cup chopped carrots	⅛ teaspoon pepper
½ cup chopped celery	1 bay leaf

1 Sort and wash the beans; place them in a large bowl. Cover with water 2 inches above the beans; let soak overnight. Drain and rinse the beans, and set aside.

2 Coat a large Dutch oven with cooking spray. Place over medium heat until hot. Add the onion, carrots, and celery. Sauté until the vegetables are crisp-tender.

3 Add the reserved beans to the vegetable mixture. Stir in the water and the remaining ingredients. Bring to a boil. Cover; reduce heat, and simmer 1 hour. Remove and discard the bay leaf. Pour half of the mixture into an electric blender or food processor; process until smooth. Return to the Dutch oven; stir well. Cook over low heat until thoroughly heated.

Tip: A stick mixer (shown in Figure 12-2) is a handy tool for this recipe. You can find them at many discount stores that sell small kitchen appliances. You'll save the time on pouring soup back and forth from the blender and have less cleanup.

Per serving: Calories 185 (From Fat 8); Fat 1g (Saturated 0g); Cholesterol 1mg; Sodium 635mg; Carbohydrate 35g (Dietary Fiber 8g); Protein 11g.

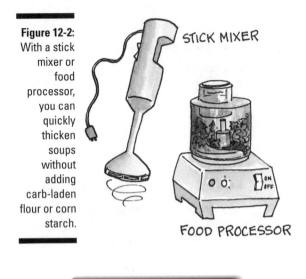

Figure 12-2: With a stick mixer or food processor, you can quickly thicken soups without adding carb-laden flour or corn starch.

STICK MIXER

FOOD PROCESSOR

Jim's Sausage Soup

Using canned vegetables in this soup makes it a breeze to prepare. You can easily make a hearty weeknight meal in under an hour. Of course, the longer it simmers, the better the flavor — but either way, this soup's a winner.

Preparation time: *10 minutes*

Cooking time: *45 minutes*

Yield: *8 servings (**1 carbohydrate choice per serving**)*

Vegetable cooking spray

16-ounce package Healthy Choice small link sausages, cut in pieces

1 medium to large onion, quartered

Two 14.5-ounce cans sliced potatoes, drained

Two 10-ounce cans diced tomatoes and green chilies

14.5-ounce can stewed Mexican-style tomatoes

16-ounce can tomato juice

Two 4-ounce cans mushroom stems and pieces, drained

16 ounces water, if needed

1 Spray the bottom of a 4-quart saucepan with cooking spray. Brown the cut-up sausages and onion.

2 Add all the other ingredients to the saucepan. Simmer for 30 minutes.

Per serving: Calories 160 (From Fat 15); Fat 2g (Saturated 1g); Cholesterol 20mg; Sodium 1,426mg; Carbohydrate 26g (Dietary Fiber 3g); Protein 9g.

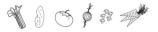

Soothing side dishes

If entrees are the main event, side dishes are a welcome distraction. Try these low-carb comfort foods to add interest to your meal and remind you of home. You can also spend a carbohydrate choice or two to add to your meal — just don't exceed your limit of five carbohydrate choices for the whole day. From fresh salads to cheesy grits, there's something for everyone in this section.

☉ Peach Salad Cups

This side dish is a great addition to any meal. It has occasionally even made an appearance on my family's dessert menu as well. Whatever use you find for it, it's sure to be delicious.

Preparation time: *20 minutes*

Cooking time: *None*

Yield: *4 servings*

2 medium to large peaches (about 6 to 8 ounces each), peeled, halved, and pitted

1 tablespoon lime juice, divided

½ cup fresh raspberries (or strawberries, quartered)

2 tablespoons unsweetened peach nectar

¼ teaspoon almond extract

1 packet of Splenda (optional)

Curly leaf lettuce leaves (optional)

1 Carefully scoop out the pulp from the peach halves, leaving a ¼-inch-thick shell. (I use a grapefruit knife to make this job a snap.) Chop the pulp, and set it aside. Brush the peach shells with 2 teaspoons lime juice to prevent browning. Set aside.

2 Combine the reserved pulp, the berries, the peach nectar, the remaining 1 teaspoon of lime juice, and the almond extract in a small bowl. Toss gently to coat. If it tastes a little too tart, add a packet of Splenda. Spoon 3 tablespoons of the peach-berry mixture into each peach shell. Serve on curly-leaf lettuce leaves, if desired.

Tip: This recipe works best with ripe, in-season peaches. You can make it ahead — just cover and refrigerate until ready to serve.

Per serving: Calories 49 (From Fat 1); Fat 0g (Saturated 0g); Cholesterol 0mg; Sodium 0mg; Carbohydrate 13g (Dietary Fiber 3g); Protein 1g.

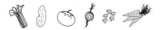

⏱ Pinto Bean Salad

This quick salad is a welcome addition to any luncheon. Make sure your cilantro is fresh, and consider throwing in more than the recipe calls for if you're a cilantro fan. Truly, you can't use too much. Season it up!

Preparation time: *10 minutes*

Cooking time: *None*

Yield: *8 servings (½ **carbohydrate choice per serving**)*

Two 15-ounce cans pinto beans

1 cup shredded Romaine lettuce

½ cup chopped celery

⅓ cup chopped purple onion

¼ cup chopped sweet red pepper

3 tablespoons red wine vinegar

2 tablespoons vegetable oil

2 teaspoons minced fresh cilantro

¼ teaspoon garlic salt

Lettuce leaves

½ cup shredded reduced-fat cheddar cheese

1 Place the pinto beans in a colander, and rinse under cold water for 1 minute. Set the colander aside, allowing the beans to drain 1 minute.

2 Combine the beans, lettuce, celery, onion, and red pepper in a large bowl; set aside. Combine the vinegar, oil, cilantro, and garlic salt in a jar; cover tightly, then shake vigorously. Pour the vinegar mixture over the reserved bean mixture; toss gently to coat well. Cover and chill thoroughly.

3 To serve, spoon the bean mixture into a lettuce-lined salad bowl and sprinkle with cheese.

Per serving: *Calories 119 (From Fat 48); Fat 5g (Saturated 1g); Cholesterol 5mg; Sodium 196mg; Carbohydrate 13g (Dietary Fiber 3g); Protein 5g.*

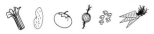

☺ *Hearty Breakfast Muffins*

These dense muffins can easily serve as a breakfast in and of themselves. They're great when paired with yogurt or string cheese for a complete meal. You'll need a candy thermometer to check the temperature of the heated milk in this recipe. And use muffin cup liners when baking these muffins.

Preparation time: *20 minutes*

Cooking time: *20 to 25 minutes*

Yield: *12 servings* **(1 carbohydrate choice per serving)**

½ **cup whole-wheat flour**	1 cup skim milk
½ **cup all-purpose flour**	½ **cup instant grits**
½ **cup cornmeal**	3 tablespoons canola oil
2 teaspoons baking powder	2 eggs, beaten
⅛ teaspoon salt	Vegetable cooking spray
½ cup chopped lean cooked ham	
½ cup reduced-fat sharp cheddar cheese, cut into small cubes	

1 Preheat oven to 375 degrees. Combine the flours, cornmeal, baking powder, salt, ham, and cheese in a large bowl; make a well in the center of the mixture. Set aside.

2 Place the milk in a small saucepan; cook over low heat, stirring constantly, until the mixture reaches 120 to 130 degrees. Cool to 105 to 115 degrees. (Use a candy thermometer to check the temperature.) Combine the milk and grits, stirring well. Combine the canola oil and eggs in a small bowl. Add the grits mixture and egg mixture to the dry ingredients, stirring just until moistened.

3 Spoon the batter into the muffin pans lined with muffin cup liners, filling each three-fourths full. Bake for 20 to 25 minutes, or until the muffins are lightly browned.

Per serving: *Calories 154 (From Fat 53); Fat 6g (Saturated 1g); Cholesterol 41mg; Sodium 313mg; Carbohydrate 19g (Dietary Fiber 1g); Protein 6g.*

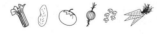

☉ Mildred's Cheesy Grits

What Southern table would be complete without grits? You can get a delicious variation on this Southern mainstay in your very own kitchen with this quick recipe.

Preparation time: *5 minutes*

Cooking time: *20 minutes*

Yield: *4 servings* (*1 carbohydrate choice per serving*)

2 cups water	Dash of garlic powder (optional)
½ cup quick grits, uncooked	Paprika
4 ounces processed cheese spread, cubed	

1 Bring the water to a boil; slowly stir in the grits. Reduce the heat; simmer 3 to 4 minutes or until thick, stirring occasionally.

2 Add the cheese and garlic powder; continue cooking until the cheese is melted, about 2 to 3 minutes. Sprinkle with paprika.

Per serving: Calories 179 (From Fat 66); Fat 7g (Saturated 5g); Cholesterol 24mg; Sodium 394mg; Carbohydrate 19g (Dietary Fiber 0g); Protein 8g.

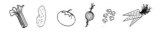

Entrees

The entrée, with its accompanying vegetables and side dishes, is the focal point of a healthy meal. These entree recipes are easy to prepare and focus on a lean protein accompanied by fruits and vegetables. Planning ahead and having ingredients ready overcomes the temptation to call the pizza delivery man or grab fast food.

Beyond fish sticks: Your Green Light guide to seafood

Fish is a delicious part of just about every healthy eating plan known to man. Quick and easy to prepare, preparing seafood can be as simple as sautéing your favorite fish with a tiny bit of olive oil and a few simple spices and finishing it with a touch of lemon. Or, if you'd rather have a recipe to follow, try one of the recipes in this section, all of which are easy to prepare.

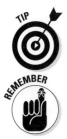

Start simple and expand your tastes. White-flesh fish (like cod, sole, halibut, and catfish) tend to be milder and are good fish to start with if you're not used to eating seafood. Work up toward fresh tuna and salmon ("fishier" fish).

Shellfish are an excellent source of protein and add almost no fat to your diet. For more on the nutritional value of seafood for a low-carb diet, see Chapter 5.

Baked Catfish Delight

Catfish is a great starter fish. Typically, this mild white fish is served fried with a side of hush puppies. You can make it low-carb-friendly with this easy recipe. Serve it with a side of light coleslaw or salad for a real treat

Preparation time: *30 minutes (plus 1 hour standing time)*

Cooking time: *50 minutes*

Yield: *4 servings*

4 catfish fillets (1 pound)	*1 clove garlic, minced*
¼ cup lemon juice	*1 small tomato, diced*
¼ teaspoon Italian seasoning	*¼ teaspoon salt*
Vegetable cooking spray	*⅛ teaspoon pepper*
½ cup green onions, chopped	*1 cup shredded part-skim mozzarella cheese*
1 medium sweet red pepper, seeded and chopped	

1 Rinse the fillets with cold water, and pat dry. Place in a shallow dish. Pour the lemon juice over the fillets; sprinkle with Italian seasoning. Cover and refrigerate 1 hour.

2 Preheat the oven to 350 degrees. Coat a large skillet with cooking spray and place over medium heat until hot. Add the onions, sweet red pepper, and garlic; sauté until the vegetables are tender, approximately 6 minutes. Add the tomato and sauté until thoroughly heated. Remove the mixture from the heat.

3 Remove the fillets from the lemon juice; place in a 12-x-8-x-2-inch baking dish. Sprinkle with salt and pepper. Bake, uncovered, for 15 minutes. Spoon the reserved vegetable mixture evenly over the fillets; sprinkle with cheese. Bake for an additional 10 minutes or until the fish flakes easily when tested with a fork.

Per serving: Calories 236 (From Fat 124); Fat 14g (Saturated 5g); Cholesterol 67mg; Sodium 323mg; Carbohydrate 6g (Dietary Fiber 1g); Protein 25g.

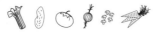

Cajun Shrimp

Charcoal grilling gives this shrimp an excellent flavor, but a gas or indoor grill or broiler will also work. Use two skewers for each kabob to keep the shrimp from spinning around independently.

Preparation time: *5 minutes (plus 15 minutes standing time)*

Cooking time: *4 minutes*

Yield: *4 servings*

3 green onions, minced

2 tablespoons lemon juice

¾ teaspoon garlic powder

2 teaspoons paprika

¼ teaspoon salt

¼ teaspoon black pepper

¼ teaspoon cayenne pepper

1 tablespoon olive oil

1½ pounds medium shrimp, shelled with tails intact, deveined (see Figure 12-3)

Lemon wedges (optional)

1 Combine the onions, lemon juice, garlic, paprika, salt, black pepper, and cayenne pepper in a 2-quart glass dish; stir in the oil. Add the shrimp; turn to coat. Cover and refrigerate at least 15 minutes.

2 Thread the shrimp onto metal or wooden skewers (if using wooden skewers, soak them in hot water for 30 minutes before use to prevent burning). Grill the shrimp over medium-hot coals about 2 minutes per side until opaque. Serve immediately with lemon wedges.

Vary It! *A quick variation is to use a bottled zesty cocktail sauce mixed with the olive oil as a marinade. Stir-fry shrimp in a skillet sprayed with nonstick cooking spray until the shrimp are opaque, just a couple of minutes.*

Per serving: Calories 168 (From Fat 45); Fat 5g (Saturated 1g); Cholesterol 252mg; Sodium 437mg; Carbohydrate 3g (Dietary Fiber 1g); Protein 28g.

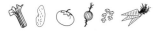

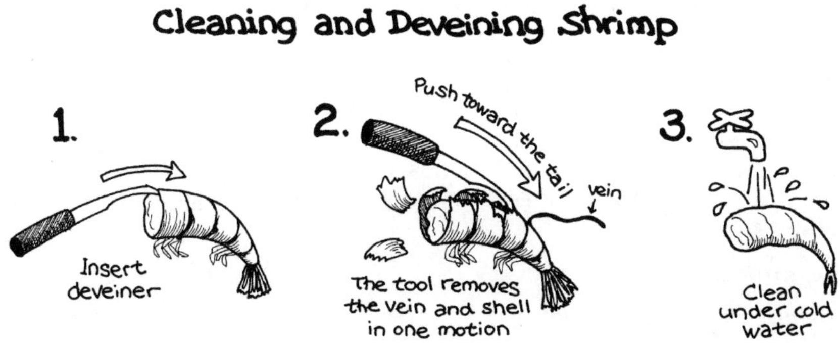

Cleaning and Deveining Shrimp

Figure 12-3:
Follow these
steps to
devein
shrimp.

1. Insert deveiner

2. Push toward the tail — vein
The tool removes
the vein and shell
in one motion

3. Clean under cold water

Onion-Lemon Fish

Use any fish (fresh or frozen) with this tasty recipe. For an extra kick, try adding a few capers with the first set of ingredients. They'll give the dish a mildly salty, slightly acidic flavor. Delicious!

Preparation time: *10 minutes*

Cooking time: *20 minutes*

Yield: *6 servings*

2 medium onions, thinly sliced

1 large lemon, thinly sliced

½ cup white wine

Small bay leaf

½ teaspoon whole peppercorns

1 cup water

1½ pounds fish fillets

1 Combine all the ingredients except the fish fillets in a large skillet and gently simmer for 10 minutes. Add the fish.

2 Cover and continue to cook 10 minutes longer.

Note: *I like to serve this fish with a quick dill sauce I whip up my self. Combine ⅓ cup plain low-fat yogurt with ½ teaspoon dried dill, plus fresh dill, if available. Let stand in the refrigerator for an hour or so to meld the flavors. Delicious!*

Per serving: Calories 102 (From Fat 11); Fat 1g (Saturated 0g); Cholesterol 53mg; Sodium 84mg; Carbohydrate 3g (Dietary Fiber 1g); Protein 19g.

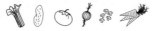

Bertie Jo's Salmon Wellington

This recipe is a particularly good choice as you begin to replace saturated fats with unsaturated fats. You're losing some saturated fat in the light cream cheese and picking up some unsaturated fat in the almonds, plus you have the heart-healthy fish oils of the salmon. Excellent! This recipe is very easy but looks very impressive to your fortunate guests.

Preparation time: *20 minutes*

Cooking time: *25 to 30 minutes*

Yield: *6 servings (**1 carbohydrate choice per serving**)*

6 salmon fillets, 4 ounces each	½ cup sliced almonds
6 ounces light cream cheese, room temperature	**½ package puff pastry**

1 Preheat the oven to 400 degrees.

2 Slice the salmon fillets lengthwise to make a pocket for stuffing if they're thick enough. If the fillets are thin, just leave them flat.

3 Mix the cream cheese with the almonds. Gently work the stuffing into the pocket of the salmon fillet. For thin fillets, spread the cream cheese–almond mixture on half of the fillet and fold the other half over it.

4 Divide the puff pastry sheet into 6 portions. Roll out to ⅛-inch thickness. Working quickly, wrap each fillet completely in the pastry dough. Seal the edges with water. Bake until the dough is browned, approximately 25 to 30 minutes.

Per serving: Calories 475 (From Fat 265); Fat 30g (Saturated 7g); Cholesterol 86mg; Sodium 292mg; Carbohydrate 20g (Dietary Fiber 2g); Protein 32g.

Chicken and beef: It's what's for dinner, and lunch, and . . .

Chicken is popular and easy to prepare. You can combine it with tasty vegetables and sauces to make a healthy meal. The chicken producers have made your culinary life easier by offering chicken in an almost endless variety of ways including individually quick-frozen pieces, boneless, skinless, marinated, pre-roasted, fresh, organic, free range . . . the list goes on. Use whatever chicken products best fit your lifestyle and budget. The more processed a chicken is, the more expensive. Find your comfort level with a balance between the two.

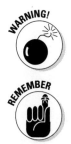

Watch out for marinated meats, including chicken, in your local grocery store. They may be convenient, but they're often *loaded* with extra sugar and salts that are completely unnecessary and very unfriendly to low-carb dieters.

Don't be afraid of lean beef. You can serve it two to three times per week accompanied by a variety of vegetables and fruits. Look for the leanest ground beef. Don't be afraid to ask your butcher or meat-department manager to trim roasts and steaks before wrapping and weighing them for you. The leaner the better, and who wants to pay for excess fat? (See Chapter 11 for more details on beef grading.)

Bertie Jo's Company Chicken

This is an easy recipe to make when you're having company over for dinner. While it's baking, you have plenty of time to attend to other dinner details.

Preparation time: *10 minutes*

Cooking time: *3 hours*

Yield: *6 servings (½ carbohydrate choice per serving)*

6 chicken breast halves, split in two	**1 can Healthy Recipe cream of mushroom soup**
3 strips lean bacon, cut in half	*8 ounces sour cream*
2.25-ounce jars dried beef	

1 Preheat the oven to 275 degrees. Lay the bacon across the chicken lengthwise. Wrap the chicken and bacon in the beef slices (one on each side); secure with toothpicks.

2 Combine the soup and sour cream. Pour over the chicken. Bake uncovered for approximately 3 hours, basting occasionally. Do not overbake.

Per serving: Calories 275 (From Fat 120); Fat 13g (Saturated 7g); Cholesterol 98mg; Sodium 671mg; Carbohydrate 5g (Dietary Fiber 0g); Protein 32g.

Eggplant Casserole

This recipe is an excellent well-rounded meal in and of itself. It has your veggies and protein all in one easy recipe. Add a green salad and light dressing for a high-fiber, filling side dish.

Preparation time: *20 minutes*

Cooking time: *1 hour*

Yield: *8 to 10 servings*

1½ pounds extra-lean ground beef	1 onion, thinly sliced
½ teaspoon rosemary	10 fresh mushrooms, sliced
½ teaspoon oregano	16-ounce container cottage cheese
½ teaspoon basil	3 eggs
1 teaspoon salt	½ pound reduced-fat Monterey Jack cheese, grated
½ teaspoon pepper	
1 eggplant	

1 Preheat the oven to 400 degrees. Brown the meat until crumbly; drain off any fat. Add the rosemary, oregano, basil, salt, and pepper. Set aside.

2 Spray a 13-x-9-x-2-inch casserole dish with cooking spray. Slice the eggplant ¼-inch thick. Quarter the slices and arrange them on the bottom of the casserole dish. Top with the meat mixture. Place the onion slices on top of the meat. Add a layer of mushrooms.

3 Beat the cottage cheese and eggs together. Spoon over the casserole. Sprinkle with grated cheese. Bake, uncovered, for 1 hour.

Per serving: Calories 241 (From Fat 118); Fat 13g (Saturated 7g); Cholesterol 105mg; Sodium 666mg; Carbohydrate 7g (Dietary Fiber 2g); Protein 25g.

Healthy salads and easy dressings

Salads are a healthy way to enjoy a variety of leafy greens and colorful veggies. Add fresh blueberries, strawberries, or raspberries for a surprising twist. Keep the dressing light to enjoy the full flavor of the greens.

South-of-the-Border Salad

Use your favorite lettuce in this easy Latin-inspired salad. Romaine is great; butter lettuce works as well. Iceberg is the traditional Americanized choice for this type of salad, but it lacks the nutrition of other lettuces. Experiment with redleaf, greenleaf, and any other varieties in your produce section.

Preparation time: *20 minutes*

Cooking time: *5 to 10 minutes*

Yield: *4 servings* **(1 carbohydrate choice per serving)**

2 tablespoons vegetable oil	2 small tomatoes, chopped
1 pound extra-lean ground beef	1 avocado, peeled and diced
1 small onion, chopped	4-ounce can sliced ripe olives, drained
3 cloves garlic, minced	**16-ounce can pinto beans, drained**
2 teaspoons chili powder	2 cups grated reduced-fat sharp cheddar cheese
½ teaspoon ground cumin	
1 head of lettuce	

1 Brown the meat and onion in the oil until the onion is translucent. Drain off the excess liquid. Stir in the garlic, chili powder, and cumin. Continue to cook 5 to 10 minutes. Set aside and let cool.

2 Tear up the leaves of lettuce. Add the tomato, avocado, olives, beans, cheese, and the meat mixture. Toss gently to mix.

Tip: *Try this great salad with different types of beans, like black beans, kidney beans, or garbanzo beans — whatever you have handy and in your pantry for a quick weeknight meal. Serve it with your favorite salad dressing and Blue Corn Crackers (see the recipe later in this chapter).*

Per serving: *Calories 509 (From Fat 316); Fat 35g (Saturated 13g); Cholesterol 71mg; Sodium 696mg; Carbohydrate 14g (Dietary Fiber 7g); Protein 35g.*

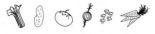

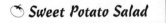 **Sweet Potato Salad**

Sweet potatoes are an excellent source of vitamin C, beta-carotene, and fiber. More importantly, they rank low in glycemic load. Eaten in moderation, they can be low-carb-friendly, because they pack such a nutritional punch.

Preparation time: *10 minutes*

Cooking time: *6 to 7 minutes (plus 2 minutes standing time)*

Yield: *4 servings* **(1 carbohydrate choice per serving)**

¾ *pound sweet potatoes, peeled and cubed*	*1 tablespoon lemon juice*
3 tablespoons water	½ *teaspoon sugar*
1 tablespoon vegetable oil	*Curly lettuce leaves*

1 Place the sweet potatoes and water in a 1-quart casserole dish. Cover and microwave on high for 6 to 7 minutes, stirring after 3 minutes. Let stand 2 minutes in the microwave. Drain the potatoes well, and set aside.

2 Combine the vegetable oil, lemon juice, and sugar; pour over the reserved potatoes. Toss gently to coat. Serve at room temperature on curly lettuce leaves.

Per serving: Calories 104 (From Fat 33); Fat 4g (Saturated 0g); Cholesterol 0mg; Sodium 9mg; Carbohydrate 17g (Dietary Fiber 1g); Protein 1g.

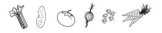

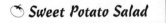 **Avocado-Orange Salad**

Don't miss this combination of the cool avocado and slightly acidic dressing. It's a great change from the typical entree salad, but the fat in the avocado makes it deliciously filling.

Preparation time: *15 minutes*

Cooking time: *None*

Yield: *4 servings*

3 tablespoons orange juice

1½ tablespoons olive oil

1 tablespoon lemon juice

Sugar substitute equivalent to 1½ teaspoons sugar

1 teaspoon Dijon mustard

½ teaspoon salt

½ teaspoon pepper

10-ounce bag mixed salad greens

1 ripe avocado, peeled, seeded, and diced

11-ounce can mandarin oranges, drained

3 green onions, thinly sliced

1 Combine the orange juice, olive oil, lemon juice, sugar substitute, mustard, salt, and pepper together in a medium bowl. Whisk in to blend and make the dressing.

2 Combine the salad greens, avocado, oranges, and onions in a large bowl. Toss gently with the dressing to coat.

Per serving: Calories 161 (From Fat 105); Fat 12g (Saturated 2g); Cholesterol 0mg; Sodium 345mg; Carbohydrate 15g (Dietary Fiber 6g); Protein 3g.

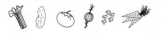

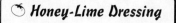

🍅 Honey-Lime Dressing

Keep this delicious dressing in the refrigerator to pour over fresh fruit any time.

Preparation time: 5 minutes

Cooking time: None

Yield: 1 cup

⅔ cup honey

⅓ cup lime juice

Combine the honey and lime juice in a clean glass bottle. Shake vigorously to mix.

Per 1 tablespoon: Calories 45 (From Fat 0); Fat 0g (Saturated 0g); Cholesterol 0mg; Sodium 1mg; Carbohydrate 12g (Dietary Fiber 0g); Protein 0g.

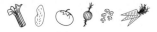

❦ Lo-Cal Salad Dressing

Make a great salad out of any bunch of fresh veggies. This terrific dressing is good with any tossed vegetable salad.

Preparation time: *5 minutes*

Cooking time: *None*

Yield: *12 ounces*

6 ounces white vinegar

6 ounces water

1 heaping teaspoon garlic salt

½ teaspoon sugar substitute

Combine all the ingredients in a dressing bottle. Shake vigorously. Store in the refrigerator, shaking well before each use.

Per 1 tablespoon: *Calories 0 (From Fat 0); Fat 0g (Saturated 0g); Cholesterol 0mg; Sodium 76mg; Carbohydrate 0g (Dietary Fiber 0g); Protein 0g.*

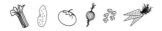

Side Dishes

Besides increasing the nutrition power in your meal, fruits and vegetables help give your meals contrast in flavor, texture, color, and shape. They also fill up your tummy without filling up your calorie and carb load for the day. Look for the freshest fruits and veggies to add the most flavor to your meals, but the canned, frozen, or dried varieties work well, too. Vary the vegetables you eat to add the most interest — sticking to any eating plan is tough if it's boring. Check out Chapter 5 for more information on how fruits and veggies can be your partners in low-carb eating.

Fruit fusion

Fruit, with its naturally sweet flavor, is a great way to spark up a meal. Use lemon slices, small bunches of grapes, or small watermelon wedges to give a simple meal immediate pizzazz. Keep fresh fruit washed and handy, so it's readily available to the whole family for quick snacking. These great recipes give you useful ideas for incorporating fruits into your diet all day long.

Sweet and Spicy Oranges

The rind of the orange gives this dish its zesty tang. The rind is the top layer of orange peel that's scraped off the outside of the orange. When you scrape the rind off the outside with a grater, avoid pushing through to the *pith* (the thick white fibrous layer before you get to the meat of the orange). The rind provides a great flavor while the pith is very bitter.

Preparation time: *20 minutes (plus standing time)*

Cooking time: *None*

Yield: *8 servings (¹/₂ **carbohydrate choice per serving**)*

8 large navel oranges	*¹/₄ **cup powdered sugar***
Few drops orange extract	*¹/₄ teaspoon cinnamon*
1 tablespoon water	

1 Finely grate the rind of 2 oranges; set the rind aside. Remove and discard the peel and pith of all oranges. Slice the oranges crosswise into ¼-inch-thick slices and arrange on a serving platter.

2 Mix the orange extract with water and sprinkle over the orange slices. Sift the powdered sugar over the top, and sprinkle with the reserved rind. Cover and refrigerate at least 2 hours. Sprinkle with cinnamon just before serving.

Per serving: Calories 80 (From Fat 1); Fat 0g (Saturated 0g); Cholesterol 0mg; Sodium 58mg; Carbohydrate 20g (Dietary Fiber 4g); Protein 2g.

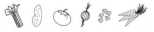

☕ Carol's Broiled Cinnamon Peaches

This recipe reminds me of peach cobbler without the pastry and is ideal for low-carb dieters. If you have an extra dairy serving left over, add ½ cup light vanilla ice cream with no sugar added. Delicious!

Preparation time: *10 minutes*

Cooking time: *5 to 10 minutes*

Yield: *8 servings*

Two 15-ounce cans peach halves canned in extra-light syrup

2 tablespoons light margarine

2 teaspoons brown sugar substitute

1 Drain the peaches. Place the peaches cut side up in a broiler pan. Dot the center of each peach with the light margarine. Sprinkle lightly with the brown sugar substitute. Sprinkle with cinnamon.

2 Broil approximately 5 to 10 minutes until browned.

Per serving: Calories 43 (From Fat 14); Fat 2g (Saturated 0g); Cholesterol 0mg; Sodium 34mg; Carbohydrate 8g (Dietary Fiber 1g); Protein 0g.

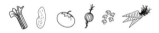

☕ Apple Treats

Dates play a starring role in this afternoon snack. Pick your favorite apple for an easy variation.

Preparation time: *10 minutes*

Cooking time: *None*

Yield: *24 slices*

2 tablespoons chopped dates

1 ounce Neufchatel cheese, softened

1 tablespoon peanut butter

½ teaspoon grated orange rind

4 medium Red Delicious apples, cored

1 Combine the dates, cheese, peanut butter, and orange rind, stirring well.

2 Stuff 1 tablespoon of the mixture into the cavity of each apple. Cut each stuffed apple into 6 slices. Serve immediately.

Per serving: Calories 23 (From Fat 6); Fat 1g (Saturated 0g); Cholesterol 1mg; Sodium 8mg; Carbohydrate 4g (Dietary Fiber 1g); Protein 0g.

 **Pimiento Cheese–Apple Wedges**

 The filling for these apple wedges makes a great dip of filling for celery as well. Try it for a quick afternoon snack or easy lunch.

Preparation time: *10 minutes*

Cooking time: *None*

Yield: *24 pieces*

2 tablespoons shredded reduced-fat sharp cheddar cheese

1 tablespoon chopped pecans, toasted

1 tablespoon diced pimiento

2 ounces Neufchatel cheese, softened

2 drops hot sauce

4 medium Red Delicious apples, cored

1 Combine the cheddar cheese, pecans, pimiento, Neufchatel cheese, and hot sauce in a small bowl; spoon evenly into the cavity of each apple.

2 Cut each apple into 6 wedges or slice crosswise into 6 slices. Serve immediately.

Per serving: Calories 24 (From Fat 9); Fat 1g (Saturated 1g); Cholesterol 2mg; Sodium 10mg; Carbohydrate 4g (Dietary Fiber 1g); Protein 1g.

Veggie power

In this section, you'll see lots of Green Light foods. So, go, go, go! Use these foods liberally.

 Cook your vegetables crisp and not mushy. Overcooking vegetables makes them soggy and causes them to lose important nutrients.

Vegetables are the true superstars of nutrition. Paired with a lean protein, they complete any meal, stave off rumbling tummies, and provide great fiber for good health.

☺ Skillet Onion Slices

This recipe is fantastic with Vidalia onions when they're in season, but you can enjoy them anytime.

Preparation time: *15 minutes*

Cooking time: *15 minutes*

Yield: *6 servings*

¼ cup low-calorie Italian salad dressing

⅓ cup water

½ teaspoon salt

3 medium onions, cut in ½-inch slices

2 tablespoons snipped parsley

2 tablespoons shredded Parmesan cheese

Paprika

1 In your largest skillet, heat the salad dressing, water, and salt. Place the onion slices in a single layer in the skillet. (Don't worry if the onions overlap a bit.) Cover and cook over low heat for 10 minutes.

2 Turn the onion slices; sprinkle with parsley, cheese, and paprika. Cook, covered, 5 minutes; cook, uncovered, 5 minutes more.

Per serving: Calories 30 (From Fat 14); Fat 2g (Saturated 1g); Cholesterol 2mg; Sodium 305mg; Carbohydrate 3g (Dietary Fiber 1g); Protein 1g.

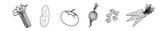

☺ Green Beans with Onions

This is a super-quick side dish that makes mouths smile. Try these green beans with Betty's Busy Day Roast earlier in the chapter.

Preparation time: *10 minutes*

Cooking time: *8 to 10 minutes*

Yield: *4 servings*

9-ounce package frozen cut green beans

½ teaspoon dried marjoram leaves, crushed

8-ounce can peeled, small pearl onions, drained

1 tablespoon tub margarine

1 Cook the beans according to the package instructions, except add marjoram to the cooking liquid. Add the onions to the beans during the last few minutes of cooking time.

2 Continue cooking until the onions are heated through. Drain thoroughly; stir in the margarine. Transfer the vegetables to a serving dish.

Per serving: Calories 54 (From Fat 26); Fat 3g (Saturated 1g); Cholesterol 0mg; Sodium 170mg; Carbohydrate 6g (Dietary Fiber 2g); Protein 2g.

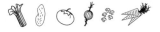

Spaghetti Squash

Spaghetti Squash gets its name from the unique way it's served. You take the cooked flesh of the squash and shred it with a fork, making it look like long threads of spaghetti.

Preparation time: *10 minutes*

Cooking time: *30 to 40 minutes*

Yield: *6 servings*

1 large spaghetti squash

Nonstick vegetable spray

3 tablespoons margarine

Salt and pepper, to taste

½ cup Parmesan cheese

1 Preheat the oven to 350 degrees. Cut the squash in half, lengthwise. Place on a baking dish sprayed with nonstick vegetable spray, cut side down, and bake until tender to the touch, approximately 45 to 60 minutes. Remove from the oven.

2 Using a fork, scrape the flesh from the cut side of the cooked squash to make "spaghetti." Continue scraping the squash to the rind. Season the spaghetti with margarine, salt, pepper, and Parmesan cheese.

Per serving: Calories 151 (From Fat 75); Fat 8g (Saturated 2g); Cholesterol 5mg; Sodium 334mg; Carbohydrate 17g (Dietary Fiber 4g); Protein 5g.

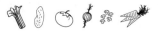

☞ Savory Carrots

You can use baby carrots in this recipe and avoid the peeling and slicing with the full-sized carrots. Pick your poison, er, I mean, carrot.

Preparation time: *10 minutes*

Cooking time: *8 to 10 minutes*

Yield: *6 servings*

¾ cup water	2 tablespoons Brummel and Brown
1 pound carrots, peeled and sliced	½ teaspoon salt
4 green onions with tops, sliced	

1 Bring water to a boil in a medium saucepan. Add the carrots and onions. Cover; cook over medium heat 15 to 20 minutes.

2 Remove from the heat; drain. Add the Brummel and Brown and salt. Toss lightly to coat with the margarine.

Per serving: *Calories 48 (From Fat 16); Fat 2g (Saturated 0g); Cholesterol 0mg; Sodium 220mg; Carbohydrate 8g (Dietary Fiber 2g); Protein 1g.*

☞ Summer Squash Medley

Despite its name, summer squash is available year-round in most parts of the country. This flavorful side dish is great with a broiled chicken breast or grilled sirloin. Add a mixed green salad for a filling nutritious meal.

Preparation time: *10 minutes*

Cooking time: *10 minutes*

Yield: *4 servings*

Vegetable cooking spray	2 small zucchini, sliced
1 tablespoon margarine	2 green onions, thinly sliced
1 large clove garlic, minced	1 cup cherry tomatoes, halved
1 small sweet red pepper, seeded and cut into strips	¼ teaspoon dried whole oregano
2 small yellow squash, cut into ¼-inch diagonal slices	¼ teaspoon salt
	⅛ teaspoon pepper

1 Coat a large skillet with the cooking spray; add the margarine and place over medium heat until the margarine melts.

2 Add the garlic; cook 1 minute, stirring constantly. Add the sweet red pepper, yellow squash, and zucchini; cover and cook 6 minutes. Stir in the onions, tomatoes, oregano, salt, and pepper; cover and cook 2 to 3 minutes or until vegetables are crisp-tender.

Per serving: Calories 62 (From Fat 29); Fat 3g (Saturated 1g); Cholesterol 0mg; Sodium 186mg; Carbohydrate 8g (Dietary Fiber 3g); Protein 2g.

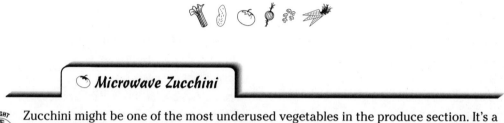

🍅 Microwave Zucchini

Zucchini might be one of the most underused vegetables in the produce section. It's a great addition to veggie trays, soups, salads, even lasagna. If you're not a fan of zucchini yet, try this very basic recipe to get started.

Preparation time: *2 minutes*

Cooking time: *6 minutes*

Yield: *4 servings*

2 zucchini	*Freshly ground pepper, to taste*
2 teaspoons margarine	*2 tablespoons Parmesan cheese, grated or shredded*
Garlic salt, to taste	

1 Wash the zucchini thoroughly. Slice each zucchini lengthwise into 2 pieces. Lay them cut side down on a microwave-safe dish.

2 Microwave on high for 2 to 4 minutes, or until barely yielding to the touch. Turn the zucchini over. Pierce with a fork, and add margarine. Sprinkle generously with garlic salt and pepper, then Parmesan cheese. Microwave about 1 minute longer.

Tip: If you ever have unexpected guests, you can quickly expand this side dish by adding more zucchini. In Step 2, microwave the batch for 1 to 2 minutes per zucchini and adjust the seasoning as desired. So for 3 zucchini, microwave 3 to 6 minutes, and so on.

Per serving: Calories 42 (From Fat 25); Fat 3g (Saturated 1g); Cholesterol 2mg; Sodium 132mg; Carbohydrate 3g (Dietary Fiber 1g); Protein 2g.

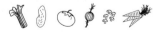

⌕ Zucchini-Tomato Bake

I go for the one-pot meal whenever possible, but this recipe is definitely worth the work. It's basically delicious Green Light veggies cooked to perfection, then topped with cheesy goodness. How can you go wrong?

Preparation time: *10 minutes*

Cooking time: *40 minutes*

Yield: *8 servings*

4 tablespoons margarine

1 onion, chopped

2 large zucchini, sliced in ¼-inch slices

3 tomatoes, chopped

¼ pound mushrooms

½ teaspoon basil

3 tablespoons chopped parsley

Garlic salt and pepper to taste

¼ cup Parmesan cheese

¼ pound reduced-fat sharp cheddar cheese, grated

1 Preheat the oven to 350 degrees. In a nonstick skillet, melt the margarine over medium-high heat. Sauté the onion and mushroom in the margarine. Add the zucchini and sauté until tender. Mix in the tomatoes, basil, parsley, garlic salt, pepper, and Parmesan cheese.

2 Place the vegetable mixture in a 1½-quart casserole dish sprayed with nonstick vegetable spray. Top with the cheddar cheese. Bake for 20 to 30 minutes.

Per serving: *Calories 142 (From Fat 88); Fat 10g (Saturated 4g); Cholesterol 12mg; Sodium 273mg; Carbohydrate 8g (Dietary Fiber 2g); Protein 7g.*

Harold's Stir-Fry

Chinese food is not terribly low-carb-friendly. With the sugary sauces and deep-fried egg rolls, it can be a diet disaster. Try this delicious alternative the next time you have a Chinese craving.

Preparation time: *20 minutes*

Cooking time: *10 minutes*

Yield: *6 servings*

2 large zucchini, sliced	1½ tablespoon olive oil
½ large green pepper, sliced	1 teaspoon powdered chicken bouillon
½ large onion, sliced	Salt and pepper
2 garlic cloves, chopped	1 roma tomato, seeded and chopped

1 Heat a nonstick skillet over medium heat until hot. Sauté the zucchini, green pepper, onion, and garlic in the olive oil. Cover the skillet, and reduce the heat to medium. Cook, stirring frequently, until the squash is barely tender, approximately 3 to 5 minutes. Do not overcook.

2 Add the chicken bouillon, salt, and pepper. Stir in the tomatoes. Cook about 1 minute more.

Vary It! *You may add 1 tablespoon of grated fresh ginger and 1 tablespoon of soy sauce for a little extra kick.*

Per serving: Calories 57 (From Fat 33); Fat 4g (Saturated 1g); Cholesterol 0mg; Sodium 164mg; Carbohydrate 6g (Dietary Fiber 2g); Protein 2g.

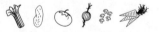

Breads, cereals, and starchy vegetables

In this section, you'll spend some of your five carbohydrate choices for the day. One of the most important components to successful long-term low-carb dieting is getting the most bang for your buck from the carbs you do eat. So look for healthy, whole-grain, high-fiber choices to satisfy your carb cravings. Don't waste carbs on processed, unnecessary sugar-laden foods that are often full of hydrogenated oils unless you just want to. Try these healthy, homemade alternatives.

☺ Hearty Whole-Wheat Muffins

These hearty muffins are worth spending some of your carbohydrate choices on. Make them ahead of time and double the recipe. Then you can always have a couple muffins for breakfast with a glass of skim milk or you can grab one from the freezer to go with that soup you made for lunch.

Preparation time: *10 minutes*

Cooking time: *10 to 15 minutes*

Yield: *12 servings* **(1 carbohydrate choice per serving)**

1 cup whole-wheat flour	¼ cup honey
1 cup all-purpose flour	¼ cup margarine, melted and cooled
2 teaspoons baking powder	1 egg, beaten
½ teaspoon salt	Vegetable cooking spray
1 cup skim milk	

1 Preheat the oven to 400 degrees. Combine the flours, baking powder, and salt in a large bowl, stirring well. Make a well in the center of the mixture. In a separate bowl, combine the milk, honey, margarine, and egg; add to the dry ingredients, stirring just until the dry ingredients are moistened.

2 Spoon the batter into muffin pans coated with cooking spray, filling each cup two-thirds full. Bake for 10 to 15 minutes or until lightly browned.

Tip: *Be careful not to overmix the batter or you'll end up with tough muffins.*

Per serving: *Calories 140 (From Fat 41); Fat 5g (Saturated 1g); Cholesterol 18mg; Sodium 221mg; Carbohydrate 22g (Dietary Fiber 2g); Protein 4g.*

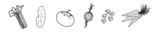

☞ Blue Corn Crackers

These crunchy crackers are a great accompaniment to the South-of-the-Border Salad in this chapter. They're a great alternative to the store-bought hydrogenated variety. Try them with tuna salad or even a hearty soup. They add crunch without the guilt.

Preparation time: *10 minutes*

Cooking time: *8 to 10 minutes*

Yield: *5 dozen small crackers, 7 crackers per serving* (***1 carbohydrate choice per serving***)

¾ cup plus 2 teaspoons blue cornmeal

½ cup all-purpose flour

¼ *teaspoon salt*

⅓ *cup margarine, softened*

¼ *cup skim milk*

1 Preheat the oven to 375 degrees. Combine ¾ cup of the blue cornmeal, the flour, and the salt in a medium bowl. Cut in the softened margarine with a pastry blender until the mixture resembles coarse meal. Sprinkle the skim milk over the cornmeal mixture, stirring just until the dry ingredients are moistened.

2 Turn the dough out onto a lightly floured surface; knead 5 to 6 times. Roll the dough to ⅛-inch thickness on a lightly floured surface; cut into rounds with a 2-inch biscuit cutter.

3 Place the rounds on an ungreased baking sheet. Sprinkle evenly with the remaining 2 teaspoons of cornmeal. Bake for 8 to 10 minutes or until lightly browned.

4 Remove from the baking sheets immediately, and cool on wire racks. Store in an airtight container.

Vary It! *For an easy variation, I sometimes brush the crackers lightly with water and sprinkle on Mrs. Dash Table Blend instead of cornmeal before baking. It's delicious and doesn't add any sodium, fat, or sugar.*

Per serving: Calories 139 (From Fat 66); Fat 7g (Saturated 2g); Cholesterol 0mg; Sodium 155mg; Carbohydrate 16g (Dietary Fiber 1g); Protein 2g.

☞ *Rye Biscuits*

Take this opportunity to expand your whole-grain horizons, with rye flour. You can find it at any natural-food store and at some larger supermarkets. If you have trouble finding it, you can substitute any whole-grain flour for the rye flour.

Preparation time: *15 minutes*

Cooking time: *12 minutes*

Yield: *12 servings* **(1 carbohydrate choice per serving)**

1½ cups all-purpose flour	*1 teaspoon caraway seeds, crushed*
½ cup medium rye flour	*3 tablespoon margarine, softened*
1 tablespoon baking powder	*¾ cup low-fat buttermilk*
¼ teaspoon salt	*Vegetable cooking spray*

1 Preheat oven to 450 degrees. Sift together the flours, baking powder, and salt; stir in the caraway seeds. Cut in the margarine with a pastry blender until the mixture resembles coarse meal. Add the buttermilk, stirring just until the dry ingredients are moistened.

2 Turn the dough out onto a lightly floured surface; knead 3 to 4 times. Roll to ¾-inch thickness; cut into rounds with a 2-inch biscuit cutter. Place on a baking sheet coated with cooking spray.

3 Bake for 12 minutes or until golden brown.

Per serving: *Calories 104 (From Fat 29); Fat 3g (Saturated 1g); Cholesterol 1mg; Sodium 193mg; Carbohydrate 16g (Dietary Fiber 1g); Protein 3g.*

☞ *Oat Bran Bread*

Bread used to be off-limits for low-carb dieters, but with this high-fiber alternative, the Whole Foods Eating Plan lets you indulge. So give it a shot, and make those Yellow Light carbohydrate choices count.

Preparation time: *45 minutes (plus approximately 1 hour 10 minutes resting time)*

Cooking time: *30 to 45 minutes*

Yield: *2 loaves, 16 slices per loaf* **(1 carbohydrate choice per slice)**

2 cups whole-wheat flour	**½ cup plus 1 tablespoon unprocessed oat bran, uncooked, divided**
1 package (.04 ounce) dry yeast	
½ teaspoon salt	**3 cups all-purpose flour**
2 cups skim milk	Vegetable cooking spray
¼ cup molasses	1 egg white, lightly beaten
2 tablespoons unsalted margarine	**2 teaspoons unprocessed oat bran, uncooked**

1 Combine the whole-wheat flour, yeast, and salt in a large mixing bowl; stir well. Set aside. Combine the milk, molasses, and margarine in a small saucepan; cook over medium heat until very warm, but not boiling (120 to 130 degrees). Remove from the heat.

2 Gradually add the milk mixture to the flour mixture, beating at medium speed with an electric mixer 3 minutes. Stir in the oat bran and enough all-purpose flour to make a soft dough. Turn the dough out onto a lightly floured surface; knead until smooth and elastic, about 8 to 10 minutes. Place in a bowl that has been coated with cooking spray, turning to grease the entire loaf. Cover and let rise in a warm place (about 85 degrees), free from drafts, 35 minutes or until doubled in bulk. (A laundry room with the dryer going works great for this purpose.)

3 Preheat oven to 375 degrees. Punch the dough down; divide into 2 portions. Cover and let the dough rest 10 minutes. Shape each portion into a loaf. Place in two 8½-x-4½-x-3-inch loaf pans that have been coated with cooking spray. Brush the loaves with egg white; sprinkle 1½ teaspoons oat bran over each loaf. Cover and let rise in a warm place, free from drafts, 30 to 60 minutes or until doubled in bulk. Bake for 30 to 45 minutes or until loaves sound hollow when tapped. Remove from the pans, and let cool on wire racks.

Per serving: Calories 92 (From Fat 10); Fat 1g (Saturated 0g); Cholesterol 0mg; Sodium 48mg; Carbohydrate 18g (Dietary Fiber 2g); Protein 3g.

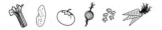

◌ Friendly Fiber Muffins

If you're trying to find ways to add more fiber to your diet, here's a great place to start. Eat these muffins for breakfast or anytime you need a filling snack.

Preparation time: *20 minutes*

Cooking time: *15 to 20 minutes*

Yield: *12 muffins* **(1 carbohydrate choice per muffin)**

Nonstick cooking spray	¾ cup skim milk
1 cup whole-wheat flour	1 egg
2 teaspoons baking powder	¼ cup honey
½ teaspoon salt	6-ounce jar baby food bananas
1¾ cups KASHI Good Friends cereal	2½-ounce jar baby food applesauce

1 Preheat oven to 375 degrees. Spray 12-cup muffin pan with cooking spray; set aside. In a small bowl, stir together the flour, baking powder, and salt. Set aside.

2 In a large mixing bowl, combine the cereal and milk; let stand for 2 to 3 minutes. Add the egg and beat well. Stir in the honey, bananas, and applesauce. Add the flour mixture and mix only until the dry ingredients are moistened.

3 Divide the batter between the prepared muffin cups. Bake 15 to 20 minutes or until lightly brown.

Per serving: *Calories 97 (From Fat 8); Fat 1g (Saturated 0g); Cholesterol 18mg; Sodium 189mg; Carbohydrate 22g (Dietary Fiber 3g); Protein 3g.*

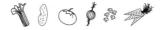

☞ *Vegetable Couscous*

This recipe can be made with just about any grain like brown rice or quinoa. Just make sure to cook the recipe to your desired tenderness and check it often toward the end of the cooking time.

Preparation time: *20 minutes*

Cooking time: *20 minutes*

Yield: *8 servings (½ carbohydrate choice per serving)*

Vegetable cooking spray

½ tablespoon olive oil

2 medium-size yellow squash, diced

1 medium-size zucchini, diced

8 small fresh mushrooms, sliced

1 small sweet red pepper, seeded and diced

¼ cup plus 1 tablespoon reduced-calorie Italian salad dressing, divided

¼ cup water

½ teaspoon salt

½ cup couscous, uncooked

1 Coat a large skillet with cooking spray, add the olive oil, and place over medium heat until hot. Add the yellow squash, zucchini, mushrooms, and sweet red pepper; sauté until crisp-tender. Combine the squash mixture and 3 tablespoons of the salad dressing in a large bowl; toss well. Set aside, and keep warm.

2 Combine the water, the remaining 2 tablespoons salad dressing, and the salt in a small saucepan; bring to a boil. Remove from the heat, and stir in the couscous. Continue to stir until all the liquid is absorbed (about 3 minutes). Add to the reserved vegetable mixture, and stir well.

Per serving: Calories 80 (From Fat 21); Fat 2g (Saturated 0g); Cholesterol 0mg; Sodium 220mg; Carbohydrate 13g (Dietary Fiber 2g); Protein 3g.

☺ Homemade Granola

Visit your local whole-foods or natural-foods market to find the ingredients for this awesome granola. You might even find that you can find the ingredients in bulk and pre-measure, buying just the amount you need. That way, when you get home, you can just dump in your bulk bags and munch.

Preparation time: *20 minutes*

Cooking time: *40 minutes*

Yield: *About 9 cups* **(1 carbohydrate choice per ¹/₂-cup serving)**

3 cups rolled oats	**¹/₂ cup rye flakes**
¹/₂ cup honey	¹/₂ cup sesame seeds
1¹/₂ cups wheat germ	1 cup hulled sunflower seeds
¹/₂ cup dry milk	1 cup raisins or other dried fruit
1 cup coarsely chopped almonds	

1 Preheat the oven to 300 degrees. Toast the oats in a 13-x-9-inch pan for about 15 minutes, stirring frequently.

2 In a separate saucepan, combine the vegetable oil and honey. Heat slowly. Stir in the wheat germ, dry milk, almonds, rye flakes, sesame seeds, and sunflower seeds.

3 Combine the honey mixture with the toasted oats and spread thinly in the pan, continuing to toast and to stir frequently another 15 minutes or until the ingredients are all toasted. Remove from the oven and mix in the raisins or dried fruit. Cool thoroughly and store tightly covered in the refrigerator. Eat dry or with skim milk or yogurt.

Per serving: Calories 287 (From Fat 119); Fat 13g (Saturated 2g); Cholesterol 3mg; Sodium 21mg; Carbohydrate 35g (Dietary Fiber 5g); Protein 11g.

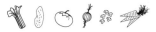

Chapter 13

Eating Out without Apologies

*E*ating away from home is so common that it's almost an assumption. A friend of mine says that when she tells her family it's time to eat, they all get in the car! Eating away from home has increased dramatically, and many people feel that you can't possibly eat out and follow a healthy diet at the same time.

In the 1950s and 1960s, eating out was rare for the typical family. When families did go out to eat, it was usually to an independently run restaurant with a variety of foods on the menu. Eating out was a very special family occasion. Today, Americans eat out more than ever before. The traditional family meal with all family members present, eating together, and leaving the table at the same time is unfortunately the exception rather than the rule. Work schedules, school schedules, sports games, band practice, and other activities have family members leaving and arriving home in different time zones. We eat in the car, at the counter, in front of the TV, and wherever else is convenient. We run errands on our lunch hour and eat snacks at our desk.

Knowing how to find healthy, low-carb options no matter where you eat is crucial. In this chapter, I tell you everything you need to know to do exactly that.

Making Smart Choices in Restaurants

If you eat out frequently, it just stands to reason that every meal can't possibly be a "treat." Instead of being "special," those away-from-home meals need to reflect how you would eat at home if you could. Why? Because when you eat at home, you have a more balanced diet. But you still need to watch portion sizes — portions at home have gotten bigger, just as they have in restaurants.

When you eat out, especially if you eat out often, you have to be more discerning in your food selections and more resistant to those restaurant marketing messages trying to get you to eat more than you need. When you eat out, enjoy being waited on and be happy you don't have to clean up, but stay in control of what you eat.

Train yourself to give the menu a more critical review and look beyond traditional entrees for food choices on the menu. Often an appetizer and soup or salad are very satisfying choices. Look for fresh fruit cups for dessert instead of loading up on rich, heavy cakes and pies.

Studying the menu

Planning ahead makes all the difference when you first begin a new dieting regimen, and choosing a low-carb life style is no exception. Create a plan *before* you order, at least until low-carb eating becomes second nature.

Make a collection of take-out menus. Every time you eat out, ask for a take-out menu. Soon you'll have menus from all the restaurants you frequent. When you aren't hungry, study the menus. Train yourself to fully examine the menu, not just pick the first thing that grabs your eye. Pizza joints have salads bars, Mexican restaurants usually have soup, and you can skip the fried rice in a Chinese restaurant. Think beyond the traditional entree. Mark items on the menu that you would enjoy eating but are also more nutritious. Look at the appetizer list. Mark the ones that aren't heavy with starch or fat. Look at the soup and salad list and then the entree items. Look for broiled, grilled, or baked items as well. Keep your balance. Look for more lean protein, fruits, and vegetables than anything else.

Go for a "test meal." Pick out a restaurant and decide you're going to make healthy choices. Use the take-out menu to pre-select your order. Bring a supportive dining partner and make your order for the healthier choice. Do the same thing at a fast-food restaurant. Go through a drive-thru and make the healthiest choice possible. The more times you do that, the easier it'll be to do it the next time.

If you aren't sure which options to choose on the menu, check out the following sections for tips on great low-carb ordering in a restaurant.

Appetizers

Select a smarter appetizer. Start your meals with a bowl of broth-based (not cream-based) soup, salad, fresh fruit, or raw vegetables. Other good choices are tomato juice, clear broth, bouillon, consommé, marinated vegetables, a fresh fruit cup, or steamed fresh seafood.

Salads

Almost any salad in a restaurant is better than no salad at all. Look for tossed vegetables, like the traditional lettuce/sliced-tomato/cucumber combo. Or protein-based dishes that include cottage cheese. If you can't be sure that the restaurant serves light or low-calorie dressings, opt for lemon juice or vinegar. And always get it on the side.

Entrees

Order roasted, baked, broiled, or grilled poultry, fish, or seafood. Look for lean meats with the fat trimmed. For more on the best lean proteins, check out Chapter 5. Order your gravy or sauce on the side. Instead of a dinner entree, consider combining a salad with a low-fat appetizer.

Vegetables

French fries are not vegetables! They used to be (in their raw form, as potatoes), but once they're peeled and fried, they lose their vegetable status. Look for raw, stewed, steamed, boiled, or stir-fried vegetables. Just about any veggie is a good veggie, until you deep-fry it, so avoid the onion rings, fried mushrooms, and so on.

Desserts

Cut back on the sweet stuff. Instead try fresh fruit or fruit juice, fat-free or low-fat yogurt, or gelatin desserts. If you must have a sweet ending to your meal, split the dessert with one or more of your friends. Order one dessert for the table and give everyone a taste.

Beverages

Go for black coffee, plain tea, sugar-free soda, or water with lemon. Avoid sugary soft drinks.

Assessing portion sizes

Restaurants are known for big portions and enticements to eat more. Value-added meals with extra-large soft drinks and fries are hard to turn down. You're better off reducing your portion size from the beginning by not ordering the large size. Recent studies indicate that people eat as much as they're served. If a regular-size burger will satisfy your hunger, but you order the jumbo burger, you'll eat all of the larger burger.

Try to keep the portion sizes appropriate. If you know the portions are too large, set some aside to take home at the beginning of the meal, not at the end. Take out the food you're reserving for later and then eat the rest.

If you've forgotten what a portion should look like, check out the guidelines for portion sizes in Chapter 4. Start measuring foods at home until you have a good understanding of a reasonable portion.

Splitting entrees

Splitting an entree with a dining partner is a good way to have a satisfying meal, reduce calories, and save money. But first ask the waiter if the restaurant allows it. Some restaurants allow you to split the entree but will bring doubles of the side items like bread or potatoes. That won't help you. Other restaurants offer half portions of the regular items.

Reducing liquid calories

Watch out for beverages. Studies show that people don't adjust their food intake for liquid calories. In other words, people don't eat less just because they're consuming extra calories in sugar-sweetened soft drinks or other beverages. Calories from beverages are purely additive to the diet. In addition to soft drinks, limit alcohol, which adds calories but no nutrition to your meal. Choose plain tea, coffee, or water instead.

Knowing how to order

Don't be afraid to ask questions about your food. You'd certainly ask questions before plunking down cash for a home or a new car. Is your body any less important or valuable?

Here are a few tips on the right questions to ask:

- ✔ If you don't know what's in a dish or don't know the serving size, ask.

- ✔ Ask for the chips or bread to be brought with the meal rather than ahead of the meal, or not at all, so you won't fill up on these items before you even see your food. Order a low-carb appetizer, soup, or juice if you're hungry.

- ✔ Ask for a fruit cup as an appetizer or the breakfast melon for dessert. Read the menu creatively.

- Confirm that you can order foods that are not breaded or fried because they add carbs and fat. If the food comes breaded, peel off the outer coating.

- Ask for substitutions. Instead of French fries, request a double order of a vegetable. If you can't get a substitute, just ask that the high-fat carb food be left off your plate.

- Offer to place your order first when eating with friends. Many people change their minds to higher calorie choices after listening to others order.

- Ask for low-calorie items, such as salad dressing, even if they're not on the menu. Vinegar and a dash of oil or squeeze of lemon are a better choice than high-fat dressings.

- Ask for fish or meat broiled with no extra butter.

- Ask for sauces, gravy, and salad dressings on the side. Try dipping your fork tines in the salad dressing, then spear a piece of lettuce. Or add a teaspoon of dressing at a time to your salad. You'll use less this way.

Making Sensible Fast-Food Selections

The average American eats in a fast-food restaurant four times a week. One popular fast-food chain has you eating out 20 times a month as its goal. High-powered advertising and enticements will be employed to help them reach that goal. What's a person to do? Raising your awareness of the situation is the first defense. Then arm yourself with good strategies to improve your food selection. Don't let someone else control your food choices.

If you're having fast food for one meal, let your other meals that day contain healthier foods like fruits and vegetables. Count your carbohydrate choices appropriately. The following sections offer fast-food suggestions.

Getting breakfast to go

If you need to stop for a quick bite before beginning your day, don't worry. Thanks to the awesome protein in an egg, most fast-food places can accommodate your diet. Choose English muffins over croissants or biscuits whenever possible; you won't get nearly the amount of fat. Order an English muffin sandwich made with egg, Canadian bacon, and cheese, and wash it down with orange juice and you'll only spend two carb choices.

Pizza restaurants

Pizza can be a good fast-food choice. Go for thin-crust pizza with vegetable toppings. Try to order by the slice. Limit yourself to one or two slices or a personal-pan pizza. If you plan for leftovers, put them away and out of sight before you dig in.

Here's one easy meal plan:

- ✓ Two slices from a 14-inch thin-crust Canadian bacon, pineapple, and veggie pizza
- ✓ Tossed salad with low-fat Italian dressing
- ✓ Diet soft drink

This makes for a delicious and filling meal, and it will only cost you two carbohydrate choices. (For more on carb choices, check out Chapter 6.)

Burger joints

Probably the most-common fast-food experience is the ever-present burger restaurant. The hamburger is the quintessential American food. Here's how you can continue to indulge, the low-carb way:

- ✓ Junior-size cheeseburger
- ✓ Kid-size or small French fries
- ✓ Side salad with low-fat dressing
- ✓ Orange juice or diet soft drink

Buffet-style restaurants

Be cautious of "all-you-can-eat" buffets or smorgasbords. The temptation to try some of everything may overwhelm your good intentions to make good food choices. Try to choose restaurants that can provide you with foods to meet your needs.

But if you do end up at a buffet table, try this trick: Picture your plate and mentally divide it into quarters. Select fruit, vegetables, and lean proteins for three-fourths of the plate. The last quarter is reserved for any starchy carbs or sweet items. See Figure 13-1 for an example of what your buffet plate should look like. Always eat more healthy foods than the less healthy ones.

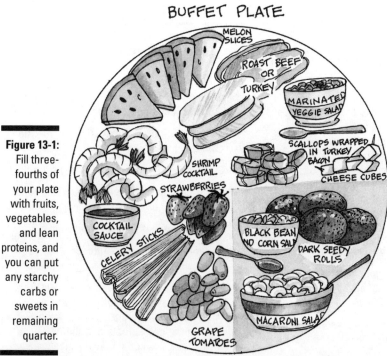

Figure 13-1:
Fill three-fourths of your plate with fruits, vegetables, and lean proteins, and you can put any starchy carbs or sweets in remaining quarter.

Evaluating Carry-Out Options

Many take-out counters in specialty food stores and supermarkets offer lightly stir-fried or roasted vegetables. This healthy indulgence costs about the same price as a high-calorie dessert. Look for fresh fruit whole or cut up. Alternately, keep fruit handy with you at all times — at home, on your desk, in your car. That way, even if the restaurant doesn't offer it, you don't have to go without.

Eating on the road or in the air

Plan a picnic at a rest stop rather than stopping for fast food. You'll be able to stretch your legs and take in some fresh air. Carry bottled water, diet colas, or fruit juice in your cooler rather than sugary soft drinks. Pack fresh fruit for snacking.

When your options are limited

If your food choices are less than ideal, don't skip the meal if you're hungry. Order regular-size portions, eat slowly, and resist the temptation to overeat. You can improve your day's food intake with healthier selections at other meals. Learn to compensate for the fast-food meal by eating plenty of fruits and vegetables at other times during the day. This tasty experience will only cost you three carb choices. If you choose to skip the fries, you'll only spend two carb choices.

Use these suggestions to improve your overall food intake in a fast-food restaurant:

- ✔ **Think about how your food will be cooked.** Chicken and fish can be good choices — but not if they're breaded and deep-fried.

- ✔ **Watch out for words like *jumbo, giant, deluxe, biggie-sized,* or *super-sized.*** Larger portions mean more calories. They also mean more carbohydrate, fat, cholesterol, and salt. Order a regular or junior-sized sandwich instead.

- ✔ **Stay away from double burgers or super hot dogs with cheese, chili, or sauces.**

- ✔ **Choose grilled or broiled sandwiches with meats such as lean roast beef, turkey or** **chicken breast, or lean ham.** Order items plain and add flavor with mustard, and crunch with lettuce, tomato, and onion.

- ✔ **Go for the salad, but watch out for the crackers and croutons.**

- ✔ **Drink orange juice and skim or low-fat milk.**

- ✔ **Order chili or soup, but no crackers.** Add the salad bar or a side salad.

- ✔ **Try coleslaw with vinegar dressing.**

- ✔ **Order extra lettuce, tomato, or other vegetables on sandwiches.**

- ✔ **End your meal with sugar-free, fat-free frozen yogurt or a small cone of fat-free yogurt.** Better yet, bring a piece of fresh fruit from home. Ices, sorbets, and sherbets have less fat and fewer calories than ice cream, but they are full of sugar. So make them a part of your carbohydrate choices if you eat them. See Chapter 6 for tips on using your carb choices for occasional treats.

- ✔ **Be alert for traps.** Fat-free muffins for breakfast may have lots of sugar.

Fresh fruit is offered at most sandwich shops, airports, mall food courts, and outdoor refreshment stands. Pack snacks when you travel, though, just in case you can't find a healthy snack. They really come in handy if you miss a flight, get stuck without an in-flight meal, or just plain don't like the food they serve.

For more on great snacks and low-carb dieting, check out Chapter 10.

Smart eating on the go

Eating smart while you're traveling can really help minimize the adverse affects of the stress that usually goes along with it. And just because you're on the go, it's not time to forget all your rules of healthy eating.

Here are some tips to keep you on the right road:

- ✔ **Practice portion control.** Try to eat the same portion as you would at home. If the serving size is larger, share some with your dining partner, or put the extra food in a container to go.

- ✔ **Eat slowly.** Your brain needs a few minutes to catch up with your stomach. Make sure you give it time to tell you you're full.

- ✔ **Reduce stress.** Find ways to reduce stress that don't involve food. (Go for a walk or do some stretches.)

- ✔ **Keep a food log and evaluate your choices against the Whole Foods Eating Plan.** Mark the food groups you're neglecting. Pay special attention to between-meal eating.

- ✔ **Be wary of impulse eating.** Today's lifestyle allows for eating any time anywhere. Keeping your food log may help you to better structure your eating pattern around your lifestyle.

- ✔ **Avoid skipping meals.** Don't skip meals — if you do, you're more likely to fill the void with snacks that provide calories, but few nutrients.

- ✔ **Reward yourself — but not with food.**

- ✔ **Eat preventively.** If you know that an eating situation will test your willpower, then eat a little snack before you leave the house — cottage cheese and fruit, a small cheese wedge and grapes, peanut butter and apple wedges, or a glass of skim milk or 100-percent fruit juice. This will take the edge off your appetite and give you better control at the eating event.

- ✔ **If your food choices were less than ideal, then compensate by choosing healthier foods at your other meals.** Remember, healthy eating is not made up of one food or one meal. It is your overall food intake that counts.

- ✔ **Exercise.** Walk off your extra food intake.

Seeing How Your Favorite Ethnic Foods Stack Up

One major reason people choose to eat out (after convenience of course) is to get a different variety of foods than they prepare for themselves at home. This doesn't have to be a license for eating to oblivion, however. Most ethnic restaurants have plenty of healthy choices.

Chinese

Authentic Chinese food features plenty of vegetables and lean meat, but watch out for deep-fried meats in sugary sauces like the one on the ever-popular General Tsao's chicken or sweet-and-sour pork. Limit your intake of the starchy, Asian-style sticky white rice. Opt for oriental noodles, like lo mein instead. Try to avoid the deep-fried foods, like egg rolls; the sweet sauces can have a lot of sugar.

Italian

Pasta dishes and bread can quickly exceed your carb limit. Thin-crust pizza with vegetable toppings is a good choice. Look for antipasto for a great selection of meats, cheeses, and marinated vegetables. It's usually on the appetizer menu. Try seafood, like savory *cioppino* (a spicy fish stew), and meat dishes, like osso bucco, braised beef shanks, or chicken cacciatore. All are great with a big salad. Skip anything parmigiana-style unless you confirm that the cutlets aren't breaded.

Mexican

Most Mexican restaurants in the United States serve high-starch, high-fat foods like refried beans, rice, enchiladas, and flour and corn tortillas. You usually start your meal with a basket of chips and salsa. The chip basket may get refilled two or three times before your food is served. These foods are denser in calories than they are in nutrients — certainly a set-up for disaster. Try sticking with grilled seafood and chicken dishes, black beans, and entrees such as fajitas. Ask the waiter to bring the chips *with* the meal instead of before. It only takes a big handful of chips to equal a carbohydrate choice.

Order bean burritos, soft tacos, fajitas, and other non-fried items when eating Mexican fast foods. Limit refried beans or ask for boiled beans. Pile on extra lettuce, tomatoes, and salsa. Watch out for deep-fried taco salad shells — a taco salad can have more than 1,000 calories if you eat the bowl!

To get you started, try this meal:

- ✔ Chicken fajitas (ask for soft corn tortillas instead of flour, and eat only two)
- ✔ Grilled peppers and onions and salsa
- ✔ Boiled beans (skip the rice)
- ✔ Tea, plain

The tortillas will cost you two carb choices, and ½ cup of beans count for one carb choice and a whopping 8 grams of fiber. For more on the benefits of fiber, take a look at Chapter 6.

Part IV
Recognizing Factors Other Than Food

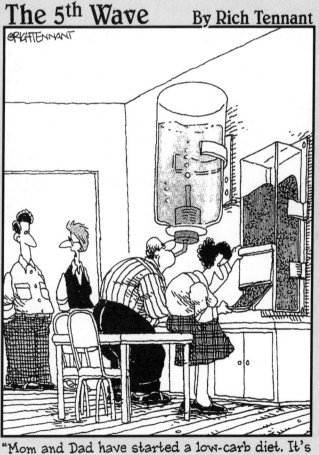

The 5th Wave   By Rich Tennant

"Mom and Dad have started a low-carb diet. It's been proven quite effective when used on hamsters."

In this part . . .

Losing weight is only part of the low-carb story. Lowering your carbohydrate intake has a whole range of health benefits, including reducing your risks of many obesity-related illnesses, like cardiovascular disease and diabetes. Exercise is an important part of any diet or weight-loss plan. In this part, I show you how you can enjoy increased energy levels, better sleeping, and reduced stress by adding exercise to your life each day. I also discuss vitamins and supplements and their role in low-carb dieting. Most of all, I help you set realistic, incremental goals for yourself, so you can look and feel great.

Chapter 14

Taking Supplements When Food May Not Be Enough

. . . .

In This Chapter

▶ Figuring out whether you need dietary supplements

▶ Understanding the ABCs of the RDA, DRI, and other fancy acronyms

▶ Choosing the right supplements for you

. . . .

The dietary-supplement industry is one of the fastest growing industries in modern times. It encompasses the manufacture and sale of vitamin, mineral, herbal, and botanical supplements. As much as 70 percent of the U.S. population is taking supplements, mostly vitamins, convinced that the pills will make them healthier and will make up for their poor eating habits. Classic vitamin deficiencies such as scurvy from vitamin C deficiency or pellagra from vitamin B_3 deficiency are almost unheard of today. But with people eating less-than-ideal diets and skimping on fruits and vegetables, marginal deficiencies are not uncommon in some groups. Marginal deficiencies in several vitamins are risk factors for heart disease, cancer, and osteoporosis.

Americans are concerned about their health and easily fall prey to advertising promising miracle health benefits by simply taking a pill. This presents a new problem to be concerned about: the dangers of excess vitamins or minerals mainly through taking too many supplements. *Remember:* There is no magic bullet; the closest thing is a healthy diet.

In this chapter, I help you determine whether you need supplements and, if so, which ones you need.

Looking First at Food

If you eat a poor diet every day, vitamins are the least of your problems. You can't replace a healthy diet with a pill. Scientists don't know what ingredient in a healthy diet is responsible for which condition. They do know that people who consume five servings or more of fruits and vegetables have less disease. Often, when the nutrients are taken out of the diet and given as a supplement instead, the person experiences no benefit and, in fact, sometimes it may even be harmful.

If there *is* a magic bullet, it's a healthy diet based on whole foods like fruits, vegetables, grains, lean meats, and dairy products. In addition to the vitamin or mineral content, whole foods contain other nutrients your body needs. Besides calcium, a glass of skim milk contains protein, vitamin D, riboflavin, phosphorus, and magnesium. Whole foods contain soluble and insoluble fiber that helps to prevent heart disease, diabetes, and constipation. Whole foods contain substances called *phytochemicals,* which help protect you against cancer, heart disease, osteoporosis, and diabetes. If you depend on supplements instead of eating a healthy diet, you miss out on the benefits of phytochemicals.

Supplements are exactly what the name implies, *supplements to* not *substitutes for* a healthy diet. Eat a healthy diet every day and then consider supplements when your health situation warrants it. Check out Chapters 5, 6, and 7 for details on what foods constitute a healthy diet.

The science of nutrition has a principle called *nutritional synergy,* which means the whole is greater than the sum of the parts. So the all-around healthy diet produces healthy results. Isolated parts of the diet do not necessarily produce isolated health benefits. Herbals and dietary supplements isolate a particular food component, but they may not provide better health benefits, because they don't have nutritional synergy. For example, people with certain types of cancer were shown to have low levels of beta-carotene and vitamin C. However, researchers were disappointed when studies showed no benefit (and even potential harm) from beta-carotene and vitamin C supplements. Beta-carotene and vitamin C are indicators of fruit and vegetable intake. Numerous studies do show that people who have diets high in fruits and vegetables have less incidence of cancer. People benefit from the nutritional synergy of a balanced, healthy diet.

Investigating Supplements

The term *supplement* describes any extra vitamins, minerals, or herbs that people take hoping to get health benefits.

Vitamins

You need vitamins for normal body functions, mental alertness, and resistance to infection. They enable your body to process proteins, carbohydrates, and fats. Certain vitamins also help you produce blood cells, hormones, genetic material, and chemicals in your nervous system. Unlike carbohydrates, proteins, and fats, vitamins and minerals don't provide fuel (calories). However, they help your body release and use calories from food.

There are 14 vitamins, which fall into two categories:

✔ **Fat-soluble:** The fat-soluble vitamins include vitamins A, D, E, and K. They're stored in your body's fat. Some fat-soluble vitamins, such as vitamins A and D, can accumulate in your body and reach toxic levels.

✔ **Water-soluble:** The water-soluble vitamins include vitamin C, choline, biotin, and the seven B vitamins — thiamin (B_1), riboflavin (B_2), niacin (B_3), pantothenic acid (B_5), pyridoxine (B_6), folic acid/folate (B_9), and cobalamin (B_{12}). There is some short-term storage of these vitamins, but because they are water-soluble, excesses of these vitamins are excreted in the urine.

Many people believe that because the excess is excreted, you can't have toxic effects from water-soluble vitamins, but this is not true. Excess amounts from supplements of some water-soluble vitamins have been shown to have negative effects.

Minerals

Your body also needs minerals. Major minerals — those needed in larger amounts — include calcium, phosphorus, magnesium, sodium, potassium, and chloride. Calcium, phosphorus, and magnesium are important in the development and health of your bones and teeth. Sodium, potassium, and chloride, known as electrolytes, are important in regulating the water and chemical balance in your body. In addition, your body needs smaller or trace amounts of chromium, copper, fluoride, iodine, iron, manganese, molybdenum, selenium, and zinc. These are all necessary for normal growth and health.

Herbs

Herbal supplements are part of a larger category of plant-derived substances known as *botanicals.* Botanicals can include bath and body products, lotions, salves, essential oils, and even insect repellent. Herbs are dried parts of plants and are usually taken to address specific health symptoms. So you may hear of people taking ginkgo biloba for memory enhancement, or St. John's wort to relieve symptoms of depression. But unlike vitamins and minerals, herbal products do not have nutritional value. They're a form of self-medication, and many people claim benefits from herbal cures. Because they're usually marketed as "natural," people tend to think of them as being safe.

Ignore the myth that herbs can't be damaging because they're natural. Most prescription drugs have their origins in natural substances and they can definitely do damage if not administered properly. High doses of ma huang (ephedra), guar gum, willow bark, comfrey, chaparral, and kava kava have been associated with harmful effects. *Do not take these herbal products.*

As of the writing of this book, there are no federal standards for herbal supplements to ensure dose, safety, or potency. Healthcare practitioners don't have a consistent agreement (with scientific fact to back it up) about what constitutes a safe and effective dose of herbal supplements. Even though some manufacturers do a good job, herbal products are not produced according to standardized guidelines and may differ in content from producer to producer. They're often marketed for a perceived drug-like effect for a medical problem but are not regulated as drugs. For more on herbal supplements, take a look at *Herbal Remedies For Dummies* by Christopher Hobbs (published by Wiley).

Establishing Your Needs

You've probably heard of the Recommended Dietary Allowance (RDA). These values provide nutrition guidance to health professionals and to the general public. They were first published in 1941 and have been updated ten times since. The original intent of the RDAs was to prevent deficiency diseases, like scurvy and rickets, in the population. However, thanks to improvements in food production and supply, vitamin deficiencies are no longer a problem in the United States. You may notice that foods like white bread and sugary breakfast cereals are *fortified* with vitamins and minerals. These vitamins and minerals are the main nutritional value you'll get from these products.

Now there is a transition underway from focusing on meeting minimum requirements to establishing optimal requirements to reduce the risk of chronic diseases such as heart disease, osteoporosis, certain cancers, and other diseases that are diet-related. Recognizing that today our problem is excess not only in calories, but also in vitamins and minerals (mainly supplied by supplements), safe upper levels of supplements need to be determined.

In 1995, a new, more comprehensive approach was developed for setting dietary guidelines. These new guidelines are called the *Dietary Reference Intakes* (DRIs). The DRIs are intended to reduce the risk of diet-related chronic conditions, establish optimal values for adults and children, and set upper levels of intake. The categories are to be determined based on strong scientific evidence. The information is released to the public in a series of reports that started in 1997 and will end in 2005.

For more information on the DRIs, see Appendix D. For the purposes of our discussion here, I'll cover the RDAs and the upper limits of what you can consume.

Avoiding Excesses

Too much of a good thing can be a bad thing, especially where supplements are concerned. Vitamin excess is definitely possible with supplementation, particularly for fat-soluble vitamins.

Because supplements aren't regulated like prescription drugs are, if you're going to move beyond the average multivitamin/mineral and calcium supplement, you must do the research to answer these questions before you begin taking the supplement:

✔ What is the upper limit for the supplements I'm interested in taking?

✔ What benefit am I hoping to achieve by taking this supplement?

✔ Will the supplement interfere with any of my other medications?

Two of the most troubling vitamin excesses occur with vitamins A and D. Excess vitamin D has been linked to hypercalcemia, which has been linked to breast cancer. Vitamin A toxicity results when excessive amounts of vitamin A supplements are consumed. Excessive vitamin A is toxic to the liver, increases your risk of osteoporosis, and may cause birth defects. So just avoid more than the RDA of Vitamin A. See the following section for the upper limits of some vitamins and minerals.

Knowing how much is too much

Because of the increasing practice of fortifying foods with nutrients as well as the increased use of dietary supplements, many people are at risk of consuming too much of certain vitamins and minerals. Scientists have determined how much is too much, and you need to be aware of these numbers so that you don't overdo it (check out Table 14-1 for the skinny on the limits). Keep in mind that these limits are based on the *total* intake of a nutrient — including what you get from food, fortified food, and supplements. It is the highest level of nutrient intake that is considered unlikely to pose any risk of adverse health effects to almost all individuals in the general population. If your intake of a given nutrient increases above the limit, then the risk of adverse effects is thought to gradually increase as well. This doesn't mean that *all* individuals will have problems at this level. It simply means that this is the level where your *risk* of developing a negative side effect increases.

If you're consistently consuming a nutrient at the upper limit, view it as a warning flag rather than a cause for alarm. Taking high levels of individual nutrients has not been shown to be beneficial for healthy people. Check with your physician, pharmacist, or registered dietitian to see if continuing to take the nutrient at the higher level is in your best interest.

Note: The ULs do not apply to anyone under the care of a physician who is taking a nutrient for medical treatment.

Table 14-1	Supplements: How Much Is Too Much	
Nutrient	*Upper Limits*	*Negative Symptoms or Reactions That May Occur Beyond the Upper Limit*
Vitamin A	More than 10,000 IU	Liver toxicity, birth defects, increased risk of osteoporosis
Niacin	More than 35 mg	Flushing (reddening of the face and/or neck accompanied by the feeling of heat)
Vitamin B_6	More than 100 mg	Loss of feeling in the arms and legs
Folic acid	More than 1,000 mcg	Worsening of vitamin B_{12} deficiency
Vitamin C	More than 2,000 mg	Diarrhea
Vitamin D	More than 2,000 IU	Hardening of the soft tissues (blood vessels, heart, lung, kidneys, and tissues around joints)
Vitamin E	More than 1,500 IU natural or more than 1,100 IU synthetic	Excessive bleeding
Calcium	More than 2,500 mg	Kidney stones, a decrease in absorption of other nutrients
Phosphorus	More than 4,000 mg	Elevated blood levels of phosphate
Magnesium	More than 350 mg	Diarrhea, confusion, depression, disorientation
Iron	More than 45 mg	Constipation, nausea, vomiting, diarrhea
Selenium	More than 400 mcg	Loss of hair and nails
Zinc	More than 40 mg	Nausea, vomiting, lower HDL ("good") cholesterol, less resistance to disease

Determining if you need more

Many Americans get most of the vitamins they need from the foods they eat, but deficiencies involving even one vitamin can lead to problems. Inadequate levels of some vitamins can lead to chronic disease, including cancer and heart disease. Also, certain medical problems can alter your need for nutrients. Here's a list of health conditions and the vitamins that may alter their progression:

- **Osteoporosis:** Vitamin D, along with calcium, has been shown to reduce bone loss and fracture risk in the elderly. For more on the dangers and prevention of osteoporosis, take a look at Chapter 7.

- **Heart disease:** Folic acid, vitamin B_6, and vitamin B_{12} may decrease risk of heart disease. Results from studies on vitamin E preventing heart disease are less conclusive. Beta-carotene (vitamin A) may raise the risk in smokers.

- **Cancer:** Lycopene, technically a non-vitamin antioxidant, may be even better than vitamin E in helping to prevent prostate cancer. It is found in tomatoes and tomato products. Folic acid has been shown to decrease risk of colon cancer in both men and women, and breast cancer in women who drink alcohol. Beta-carotene may increase risk of lung cancer in smokers.

- **Birth defects:** Folic acid appears to reduce the risk of spinal birth defects in infants whose mothers take these supplements. Excessive vitamin A during pregnancy may cause negative side effects.

- **Macular degeneration:** A common cause of vision loss in senior adults is age-related macular degeneration. Recent studies indicate that supplements of vitamin C, vitamin E, beta-carotene, zinc, and copper may slow the progression of the disease. Also, the phytochemicals lutein and zeaxanthin may prevent it. Because supplements of these nutrients can exceed recommended levels, you should check with your eye-care professional before taking them. Too much lutein can block the effects of lycopene, a phytochemical important in lowering cancer risk. Generally, people who have a lifelong habit of eating spinach or collard greens five or more times per week are almost 90 percent less likely to develop macular degeneration. If you have a family history of macular degeneration, start incorporating these vegetables into your diet.

- **Diabetes:** All essential nutrients are important in diabetes. A well-balanced diet is the very best source of these nutrients for people with diabetes. A multiple vitamin-mineral supplement may also be helpful. Check with your physician, registered dietitian, or certified diabetes educator before taking any additional supplements.

- **Homocysteine:** Homocysteine is a factor in your blood that has been recognized as a risk factor for cardiovascular disease. High levels of homocysteine are predictive of adverse cardiac events in people with established coronary artery disease. The B-complex vitamins B_6, B_{12}, and folic acid can lower homocysteine levels and reduce your risk of adverse events. Check with your physician, cardiologist, or registered dietitian to see if these supplements would benefit you.

✔ **Hypertension:** Persons taking medication to lower their blood pressure *may* need a potassium supplement. Your physician should determine whether you need one. Foods supplying the nutrients potassium, magnesium, calcium, protein, and fiber have been shown to lower blood pressure. Supplements of these nutrients do not lower blood pressure.

✔ **Lactose intolerance:** Lactose intolerance is a condition in which a person lacks the enzyme *lactase* to digest the milk sugar, lactose. People who are lactose-intolerant learn to avoid the intake of dairy foods. It is recommended that persons with lactose intolerance take a 600 mg calcium supplement one or two times per day to supplement their diet.

The elderly, vegans, and alcoholics are especially at risk for inadequate intake of some vitamins. Supplements are often recommended for these persons, but they should also try to increase their dietary sources if possible. Look for the listed natural sources to get the following vitamins:

✔ **Folic acid:** Dark green leafy vegetables, whole grains and fortified grain products, beans, avocados, bananas, orange juice, and asparagus

✔ **Vitamin B$_6$:** Fish, poultry, legumes, whole grains, nuts, peas, and bananas

✔ **Vitamin B$_{12}$:** Fish, meat, poultry, eggs, and dairy products (If you are a vegan and do not eat animal products, you will need to take a supplement of vitamin B$_{12}$.)

✔ **Vitamin C:** Citrus fruits, such as oranges and grapefruits, strawberries, melons, tomatoes, green and red peppers, and broccoli

✔ **Vitamin E:** Margarine, nuts, vegetable oils, wheat germ, and whole grains

Navigating the Sea of Supplements

With about 29,000 brands of multivitamins and antioxidants currently on the market, how do you know which to choose? Follow these guidelines:

✔ **Choose a broad-spectrum supplement that contains vitamins *and* minerals.** It should supply 100 percent of the daily value for about ten vitamins and four or five minerals. Look for vitamin A, beta-carotene, vitamin C, vitamin D, vitamin E, sometimes vitamin K, B-complex vitamins, like thiamin (B$_1$), riboflavin (B$_2$), niacin (B$_3$), pantothenic acid (B$_5$), pyridoxine (B$_6$), cobalamin (B$_{12}$), and folic acid. Look for the minerals iron, zinc, calcium, and magnesium.

✔ **Choose a calcium supplement separately.** It's difficult to get the daily amount of calcium you need in a multivitamin. If you could, the pill would be so large you couldn't swallow it. Buy your calcium as a separate supplement.

✔ **Consider gender-specific or age-specific vitamins.** Multivitamins are marketed for everybody, but with new information on requirements, you may want to choose a product specifically formulated for men or women, or for people in your own age group, including teens, children, and people over 50. The amount of iron recommended for younger women is not recommended for men or postmenopausal women. Women typically need more calcium than men. Older women need more calcium than younger men. The list goes on, but the closer you can get to your gender and stage of life, the more likely you'll find a multivitamin that fits your needs.

✔ **Save your money.** Price is not an indicator of quality. Go for the lowest-price brand available. Generic or store brands available in large national chain stores are usually modeled after popular brands and are less expensive. Compare the ingredients. They're often the same or nearly the same.

✔ **Avoid gimmicks that increase the price by including herbals and antioxidants in many multivitamin formulations.** Herbal supplements are not essential for human nutrition and may have drug-like qualities. Besides, studies show that less than half of herbal supplements sold in the United States contain the amount of potency on the label.

✔ **Watch out for marketing hype such as claims of "high potency."** There is no legal definition of such terms.

✔ **Pay attention to expiration dates.** Supplements can lose potency over time especially in a hot and humid climate. Don't buy supplements that do not have an expiration date. And obviously don't buy supplements with an expiration date if they're already expired. If you find expired supplements on the shelves, turn them in to the store manager.

✔ **Look for "USP" or "ConsumerLab.com" on the label.** The USP seal or ConsumerLab.com seal ensures that the supplement:

- Actually contains the ingredients that it states on the label

- Contains the stated amount of those ingredients

- Will dissolve or disintegrate effectively so it will release the nutrients and it can be absorbed

- Has been screened for the contaminants like pesticides and bacteria

- Has been manufactured in sanitary conditions

These seals don't mean the claims are proven or that the product has been FDA approved. It also doesn't mean that by taking this product you don't have to eat well. It just means that the product is what it says it is, not that it does what it says it does.

If you have difficulty swallowing vitamins or other pills, ask your doctor if a chewable or liquid form might be better for you. Children's chewable vitamins include adult dosing and RDA information right on the label. Calcium supplements are now available in chewable delicious flavors, like chocolate, caramel, and mochaccino.

Store supplements in a safe place and keep them out of the sight and reach of children. Lock them in a cabinet or other secured location. Be especially careful with supplements containing iron. Iron overdose is a leading cause of poisoning deaths among children.

Check with your doctor, pharmacist, or registered dietitian before taking anything other than a standard multivitamin/mineral supplement of 100-percent daily value or less. This is very important if you have health problems or are taking prescription medications. High doses of niacin can result in liver problems. An excess of vitamins E and K can interfere with blood-thinning medications such as anticoagulants and complicate the proper control of blood thinning. If you're already taking supplements and haven't told your doctor, discuss it at your next visit.

Although there are special conditions for some people that indicate a vitamin/mineral supplement, a well-balanced diet is still the best source of all essential nutrients. If supplements are indicated, they are to *supplement* the well-balanced diet not *substitute* for a well-balanced diet. Fix your diet first; then decide if you need to supplement.

Chapter 15

Setting a Fitness Goal

*B*eing healthy and fit is its own reward. To wake up rested, ready to start your day, with plenty of energy and feeling good about yourself is the foundation of a balanced healthy life. But so often, people tie all their efforts to eat well and exercise to a number on a scale or to a particular body shape. In this chapter, I help you to step back and appreciate other factors of good health, in addition to healthy weight.

If you're like most people, you may not think very much about what you eat. You get hungry and you eat until you're full. Pretty simple, right? However, the foods you choose to eat are very important in determining how you feel. Your food choices make a big impact not only in how much you weigh, but on how much energy you have, your mood, your risk of illness, and even your mental alertness. Eating well is not a test of your willpower over junk food. Eating well is a *choice* to eat foods that nourish your body, feed your cells, and allow your body to repair and heal itself. This doesn't mean never eating foods you enjoy. It means selecting foods that balance your nutritional needs.

Your diet may be the greatest individual factor affecting your overall health and quality of life.

Setting Realistic Expectations

Most people have an unrealistic view of what they should weigh. You may feel a certain amount of excitement when you go on a diet. You begin to have visions of what you weighed in high school and set out to lose 50 pounds. You may lose 20 pounds and feel like a failure because you didn't lose the other 30. But you lost 20 pounds! Who said you had to lose 50? You should congratulate yourself for losing 20 and vow to keep it off.

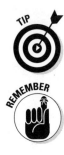

Be patient in your expectations. Concentrate on eating well and getting more exercise and don't worry about the weight loss. People respond to weight loss in different ways. The minute some people alter their diet, they drop several pounds. Other people may need several weeks before they show a weight loss.

Most early weight loss, regardless of when it occurs, is water loss. The loss in body fat starts after a couple of weeks. The more overweight you are when you start a weight-loss plan, the greater your initial weight loss will be. It isn't unusual for a very obese person to drop 10 to 20 pounds in three weeks. But he or she won't continue to lose at that rate. A healthy and more permanent weight loss is 1 to 2 pounds per week. The closer you are to your ideal weight, the slower your weight loss will be. If you have only 10 pounds to lose, your weight loss may average only ½ pound per week. However, benefits such as more energy, better sleep, and better mood happen right away.

Accepting your size

Healthy and fit people come in all shapes and sizes. But most people measure their health in numbers — the number on the scale, or the number of calories or fats or carbs they've eaten.

You're a human, not a number. You can eat well, get regular exercise, and still be larger than average. And you're far healthier than your thin counterpart who eats poorly and is sedentary. Unfortunately, society judges the thinner person as healthier than you.

Rise above the propaganda and be proud of who you are. In accepting your size, don't accept poor eating habits and inactivity. Everyone deserves a healthy diet and the chance to be physically fit. If you're overweight, you're eating too much carbohydrate. If you adjust your carbohydrate intake by lowering your *refined* carbohydrate intake, you'll lose weight, gain more energy, improve your mental outlook, and gain better health. If you stay with it long enough, you'll lose weight until your body achieves a weight that is best for you.

Understanding genetics and their effect on your body shape

Choose your parents well, because the link between genetics and health is a powerful one. In Chapter 4, I talk about the importance of knowing your family medical history. Not only are some medical problems passed down through the family, but physical characteristics are passed on as well. You don't even have to know the details to gather some important information. Look around your family and see what body shape is most common; chances are, you look like your family looks. This doesn't mean you can't counteract the genetic hand you're dealt. All body types can become overweight and all body types can become fit.

Some people are genetically predestined to be tall and lanky, round and soft, muscular and strong — and most people are a lot of variations in between. Muscular and strong is the politically correct body type that we all want to be, but that's not how it is. No matter how hard they try, round and soft will never make tall and lanky and neither type will be muscular and strong. Their muscular form is predetermined. Even though you can and should strengthen the muscle mass that you do have, there will be a genetic limit to what you can achieve. A person with a tendency to be round and soft can be extremely fit and healthy even though he doesn't have that perfect-looking body. Develop an understanding of the uniqueness of your own body and then devise a fitness plan that suits it.

Establishing Benchmarks Beyond the Scale

The scale is a mechanical device, but most people let it determine their health and their self-worth. Take ownership of your own personal body and discover what makes it feel good and what makes it feel bad. Use your waistline to judge if you're gaining or losing weight. If your clothes are tight and uncomfortable, lose weight until they fit.

You won't be able to get completely away from the scale, but don't let it be the only measure of your progress. The scale is useful to assess your weight and to measure your progress. It's normal for weight to fluctuate 3 or 4 pounds during the course of the day. Fluid retention can greatly affect your weight on the scale.

Use the scale as one source of assessment, but not the total assessment. Here are some tips:

- ✔ **Do not weigh every day or even once a week if you can avoid it.** If you do weigh daily, accept small fluctuations in weight.

- ✔ **Weigh first thing in the morning, after you go to the bathroom, and before you dress.** Try not to weigh again for a couple of weeks unless you find it useful.

- ✔ **Do not compare weights on different scales.** You're dooming yourself to disappointment. The scale in your bathroom, the doctor's office, and the gym will not synchronize.

✓ **Do not compare weights from different times of day.** You naturally weigh less in the morning and steadily gain through the day as you drink and eat. You don't instantly get fatter, but you ingest several pounds of liquid and food each day.

✓ **Don't expect your weight to maintain an exact number all the time.** It's normal for your weight to fluctuate a few pounds. Having a salty meal like pizza one night can contribute to water retention and cause you to gain a pound or two, even if you've followed the plan. You'll notice the water weight disappear in a day or two if you follow the plan.

✓ **Forget the actual number on the scale.** The main purpose of the scale is to tell you if you're gaining weight, staying the same, or losing weight. Use other measures besides the scale to evaluate your progress. Look for improvements in blood pressure, blood sugar, cholesterol levels, less hip and knee pain, or easier breathing. Look for improvements in the quality of your life, such as more energy, better sleep, better mood, and more self-confidence.

More energy

If you want more energy:

✓ Lower the total amount of refined carbohydrate in your diet.

✓ Eat less food but more often; avoid skipping meals and heavy dinners.

✓ Enjoy a variety of exercise, including strength training.

✓ Adopt a healthy, self-promoting attitude.

Better sleep

Diet factors can interfere with sleep. A big meal at night causes your body to stay up digesting it just when you want your body to calm down. Blood gets directed away from the brain and into the digestive tract, and that can interfere with sleep. Diets low in iron, calcium, and magnesium can cause poor sleep. Avoid caffeine at least four to six hours before bedtime if it is a problem for you. Caffeine is a stimulant and is found in coffee, soda, tea, chocolate, and some over-the-counter medicines. Yes, carbohydrates can increase serotonin levels which can contribute to sleep, but it doesn't have to be crackers — a piece of fruit or a glass of skim milk will do the same thing. The milk also contains an amino acid that some studies show helps people go to sleep.

If frequent trips to the bathroom are disturbing your sleep, drink less water two to four hours before bedtime. Although drinking lots of fluids is healthy, it shouldn't disturb your sleep. You need 6 to 8 glasses per day and that includes the water in fruit, soups, and other foods.

Improved mood

Eating a well-balanced diet and exercise makes your body feel good. Your body is able to thrive on the good nutrients you're feeding it because it isn't being diverted into handling excessive processed foods and unhealthy fats. When your body feels good, you feel good all over and it translates into a better mood. You're sleeping well and you feel rested when you awaken in the morning. You have more energy, which automatically gives you a more positive mental outlook.

More self-confidence

As you gain control of your eating and start exercising you will be able to gain control of other aspects of your life. This results in more confidence. Praise yourself for the healthy choices you make throughout the day. Don't focus on an occasional slip-up.

Getting Up and Moving

About 50 percent of American adults are not sufficiently active in their leisure time to achieve health benefits, and nearly 30 percent are not physically active at all.

Lifestyles today are not conducive to a lot of physical activity. We're active, but not *physically* active. Today you can drop off the kids at school, drop off the dry cleaning, deposit your paycheck, pick up your medicine, pick up lunch, and never get out of the car until you're back at home.

Here are some ideas for making those errands add up to true physical activity:

- ✔ **Park farther from the school and walk the kids to the door.** If the kids are too big to be seen with Mom, you can still park farther away and let them walk. (Activity: 10 minutes)

- ✔ **At the cleaners, park farther away and carry the clothes inside.** (Activity: 3 minutes)

- ✔ **At the bank, park outside and walk inside to do your banking.** (Activity: 3 minutes)

- ✔ **At the pharmacy, park outside and walk in to pick up the prescriptions.** Those prescriptions are all probably for something that walking will help. Get the best remedy around: exercise! (Activity: 3 minutes)

If you follow these tips, you gain a total of 19 minutes of physical activity, just in running your daily errands. That's almost one-third of the 60 minutes of activity you need to get in each day, just making a few small changes.

If you're thinking, "This will take so much time!" Well, what are you going to do with that extra time? If you'd instead use the time to go to the gym or take a walk, by all means do it. But if you're going to watch TV, talk on the phone, or do other activities that aren't so active, at least work these ideas into your lifestyle part of the time.

If you really do have a time crunch, divide up the errands. Who says they have to be done at the same time? Do part of them when you take the kids to school and the other part before you pick them up in the afternoon.

Everyone is different and each person has different demands on his or her time. So what works for one person may not work for another. The point is to take a look at your lifestyle and find ways to be more active. That's often a lot more practical than finding the time to go to the gym for an hour.

Knowing how much exercise is enough

In 1996, the Surgeon General recommended 30 minutes of exercise five times a week. But in 2002, the Institute of Medicine Dietary Reference Intake (DRI) report recommended 60 minutes of moderate intensity physical activity *every* day of the week. These guidelines are for an average-weight person. If you're overweight, first decide how active you currently are and then increase from there. Let 30 minutes of total exercise be your first goal, and when you're comfortable doing that, increase to 60 minutes as your second goal.

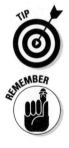

The most practical way to achieve 60 minutes of exercise is to incorporate it into your daily activities and let it add up.

Getting sufficient exercise helps with the control of your appetite. People who exercise regularly report 39 percent fewer cravings for fat and 22 percent fewer cravings for sugar than inactive people. Getting enough exercise also gives you more energy. If you're tired all the time, try a ten-minute walk. A ten-minute walk can refresh and energize you better than a ten-minute nap. And if you take walks regularly, it will give you more energy overall.

Accumulating exercise and letting it add up

Research shows that your exercise activity can be cumulative. In other words, two 15-minute walks can equal one 30-minute walk. With the new guidelines recommending 60 minutes of exercise, you need to develop a more active lifestyle overall and find ways to build exercise into your daily activities. Start maximizing opportunities in your life to move more. Small changes can add up to large increases in your daily activity level.

Here are just a few ideas to get you started:

✔ **Walk, run, and play actively with your children or grandchildren.** A good tickle session can get your heart rate up.

✔ **Mow your yard using a push mower.** If you have a self-propelled mower, alternate between using this feature and just pushing it with good old-fashioned elbow grease. If you don't have the option to turn it off, add ankle weights for an extra strength-training push.

✔ **Take the stairs instead of the elevator.** Even just a few flights a day can make a huge difference. Spend five minutes of your lunch hour going up and down to get your heart rate up in a hurry.

✔ **Clean your own house.** You'd be surprised how many calories you can burn this way. Depending on your weight and age, you could burn 200 to 350 calories per hour with this activity. Put on upbeat music while you clean. Boogie between bathrooms and salsa through the kitchen. Just keep moving. Sing as you go and you might not even notice you're working.

✔ **Wash your own car.** Do some extra detailing and maybe waxing to get some extra activities in.

✔ **Take up dance — ballroom, square-dancing, line dancing, clogging, you name it.** Most of us love music, and it's fun!

Whatever you do, do something!

Inactive, physically-unfit people have the highest death rate. Studies indicate that as physical activity increases, the death rate decreases. Robert Sweetgall, America's leading advocate of walking for fitness, gives this rundown on how much you can improve your chances:

✔ Just rising off the couch and walking 1 mile per day (2,000 steps) significantly drops the mortality rate.

✔ Increasing to 2 miles of walking per day (4,000 steps), you continue to benefit from walking.

✔ Increasing to 3 miles per day (6,000 steps) continues to lower the mortality rate to near an optimal level.

✔ Increasing beyond 3 miles per day — say to 5 miles per day (10,000 steps) — helps reduce the mortality rate a bit more. However, the primary benefits are reached in going from 0 to 3 miles per day!

Turn off the television! A recent study found that for each two hours per day increase in time spent watching television, there was a 23 percent increase in obesity risk. You won't be bombarded with food commercials and you may be surprised at how much more time you have. Use that time to be more active.

Walking your way to fitness

Walking is one of the easiest ways to add physical activity to your day. It's simple, convenient, and almost everyone can do it. It requires comfortable, but not special, clothes and a sturdy pair of walking shoes.

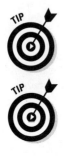

Dress for the weather. Wear layers that will allow you to cool off or warm up as needed. Take sunscreen, a hat, a water bottle, keys to your house, your ID, and maybe a cell phone.

Choose walking shoes with a low, rounded heel, a flexible sole, and plenty of toe room. They should support your arches and cushion your feet. Look for shoes that are lightweight and ventilated. Walking shoes do not have to be expensive. Shop at a discount shoe store or look for markdowns at department stores. Last season's shoes walk just as well as the latest model. Wear your shoes only for walks — not as your everyday shoes — to help them last longer.

Keep safety in mind. Choose streets with level sidewalks, a park with a well-worn path, or even an outdoor track at a local school or college. If you walk at night, walk with a companion. Make sure the area is well lit. Wear light-colored, reflective clothing or shoes to make you more visible to drivers. Skip the headphones and turn off the cell phone so you can hear traffic. Stay aware of your surroundings.

For indoor walking, look for malls, museums, or convention centers. Look at the place where you work. Walk to your coworkers' desks instead of using e-mail or the phone. Take the stairs at work and in public buildings.

Try using a pedometer not only to measure your walking, but also to motivate yourself to walk more. A *pedometer* is a pager-sized device worn on your belt that simply records the number of steps you take based on your body's movement. It's ideal for people who simply can't find 30 minutes, or even three 10-minute blocks of time, in a day for walking.

Fitness for Life: It's Never Too Late

Do you know the saying, "Today is the first day of the rest of your life"? Don't bemoan the fact that you haven't had the healthiest lifestyle. Start today and begin reaping benefits. You may be suffering consequences from poor habits in the past, but why add to that load?

Studies show that elderly people confined to wheelchairs or on walkers can improve their strength, stamina, and endurance with regular exercises. Some in wheelchairs can move up to walkers and some using walkers can switch to canes.

Step up the workload as you get older. The 30-minute mall walk you've faithfully trekked three times a week may not cut it any more. Because your metabolic rate is slowing down, you'll need 45 to 60 minutes of aerobic activity four or five times a week to reduce your body fat. Or better yet, if you're younger, get rid of the fat now, so you'll just need to maintain (rather than reduce) as you get older.

Middle-aged and older people of today grew up in a very youth-oriented society. It's often difficult for them to accept the fact that they are aging. Some people do some bizarre things to hold on to their youth and usually end up looking foolish. But why hold on to the past? Today, aging is the new "prime of life." The over-50 crowd is breaking all the rules (just like they did in the '60s) for growing older but not old. They are the role models for the future generation and are making aging an enviable state to be in. To join this "hip" crowd, change the way you think about food, fitness, and your own body image.

Start by adjusting your attitude:

✔ **Act your age.** That is to say, accept yourself and your age and move forward, not backward. One day you will see the age you are today as being very young. Don't waste it by thinking of yourself as old.

✔ **Remember that fitness is the goal — forget about being "thin."** In fact, the more meat on your bones in the form of lean, toned muscle, the higher your metabolism, which means the faster you'll burn calories. And no matter what you weigh, the more muscle mass you have, the better off you are.

✔ **Forget the scale as your primary assessment tool.** Concentrate on how you feel in your clothes.

✔ **Focus on progress not perfection.** Celebrate minor victories, like every improvement on your BMI rating. Or start smaller: Celebrate the first week you stay within your five carb choices every day. Find something to celebrate every week. Don't dwell on setbacks. Learn from them and move on. (Check out Chapter 18 for more tips on getting back on the healthy-eating horse.)

✔ **Empower yourself.** Remind yourself that you have the power to improve your health — whatever your age.

Then begin adjusting your plate:

- ✔ **Eat smaller meals, several times a day.** Afraid of between-meal snacks? Just make smart choices and you're on your way to healthy eating. Eat smaller portions more frequently to help burn more for energy and store less as fat. Never skip meals; it's energy draining and can lead to bingeing.

- ✔ **Enjoy a power lunch.** Make lunch the main meal by enjoying some of your carb choices for the day, and taper off in the evening. Try to stick to mostly Green Light foods as the day progresses. (For more on Green Light foods, check out Chapter 5.)

- ✔ **Remember that variety is the spice of life.** Choose from the different food groups, fruits, vegetables, lean protein, and low-fat dairy.

- ✔ **Don't give up your favorite foods.** Allow yourself an occasional indulgence.

- ✔ **Drink more water.** Drink at least 6 to 8 glasses a day. Try to carry a water bottle wherever you go (in your car, at your desk, in your diaper bag, and so on) so that you'll always have it with you.

Adjust your workouts by:

- ✔ **Extending your cardio workout.** By spending just five more minutes at your peak exercising rate, you can burn more calories per workout. That's a good investment in your own good health.

- ✔ **Trying strength training.** This can be as simple as adding ankle or hand weights to your walk, or as complicated as working with a personal trainer to develop a personalized plan. Wherever you start, strive to work up to at least two sessions each week. Each session should last 30 to 40 minutes. Building muscle mass helps improve your metabolism, helps you lose weight, and slows or prevents bone loss as you age.

- ✔ **Varying your activity.** Try walking, swimming, golf, whatever activity sounds fun to you. Even if walking is your only cardio activity, you can vary where you walk, and whom you walk with. Walk with your dog. Walk with friends. Walk with ankle or hand weights. You get the picture.

- ✔ **Remembering that patience is a virtue.** Don't expect to be able to do 60 minutes each of the first 7 days you start the program. Aim for every other day for the first few weeks, and then increase from there. Don't burn out or get so sore that you're unable to maintain the activity. Remember this is a marathon, not a sprint, so take it slow, but be consistent. You may not lose inches right away or drop a pant size. Those tangible improvements will take a few weeks. However, benefits in energy level, stress relief, and mood can happen during the first week.

Part V
Sticking to the Plan

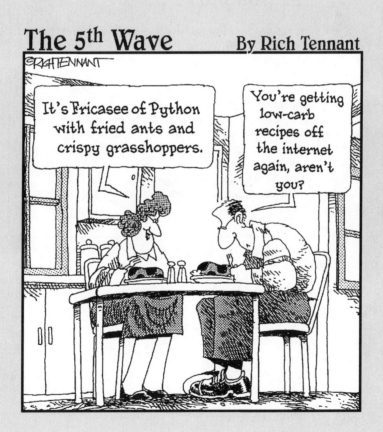

In this part . . .

As with making any long-term change to your diet, the key to enjoying the ultimate benefits is sticking with the plan. This part is loaded with tips and tricks to help you set yourself up to succeed with a low-carb lifestyle. The first step in making the low-carb commitment is mental or psychological. I show you how to psych yourself up and customize your food habits to meet the demands of your lifestyle *and* your low-carb diet. I also help you organize your pantry and your fridge to make low-carb dieting second nature — and I show you how to forgive yourself when it's not. I help you analyze what went wrong in your plan and show you how to get back on the horse, er, I mean diet.

Chapter 16

Psyching Yourself Up

. . . .

In This Chapter

▶ Developing the right frame of mind for change

▶ Assessing your level of commitment

▶ Knowing your own behavior

▶ Building a support network

. . . .

A healthy diet isn't complicated — it's a matter of choice. You've probably thought about eating healthier, exercising more, and getting more fit before, but for some reason you never seem to get there. Maybe you haven't thought the process through thoroughly enough, or maybe you've tried to do a complete overhaul of your life when making small steps would be better. Whatever the reason, today you have the opportunity to make a permanent, lifelong change. Read on!

Preparing Your Mind

Analyze your motivation by writing down every benefit you can think of for changing your diet. Is it to lose weight? Is it to have more energy and feel better? Is it to improve a problem with your health? Think of every possible reason. These are *your* reasons and not someone else's. No benefit is too small or insignificant if it's important to you.

Pick out two or three reasons that are the most important to you. Write them down on slips of paper and put them in places where you can see them every day — on the mirror, on the refrigerator, in your purse or billfold, or in a drawer at work. Review them every morning when you get up, every evening before going to bed, and several times in between. Stay focused and you will achieve your goal.

Ask yourself:

  ✔ Why am I doing this?

  ✔ For whom am I doing this?

  ✔ What are my expectations from doing this?

Visualizing Your Success

Take five minutes every day to visualize how you want to live your life. Develop a mental image of yourself being healthy and making the right choice. Think about the following images:

- Imagine yourself feeling well — alive, healthy, energetic — looking forward to each day.

- See yourself going about your daily activities accomplishing your work and feeling good about it.

- Imagine yourself selecting fruits, vegetables, lean proteins, and low-fat dairy foods because you *want* to not because you *have* to.

- Think about how good the food tastes and imagine healthy nutrients feeding your cells and nourishing your body.

Recognizing Your Level of Commitment

If you've followed the recommendations in the first two sections of this chapter, then you're well on your way to making important lifestyle changes. However, to fully establish your commitment to making changes, you need to understand your readiness for taking serious action.

In making your commitment to change, it's helpful to understand how ready you are to make the change. Researchers James O. Prochaska and Carlo C. DiClemente developed a Stages of Change model to help assess your readiness or someone else's readiness for making changes. They've identified five stages to change: pre-contemplation, contemplation, preparation, action, and maintenance. Read the descriptions of the stages in the following sections, and determine your level of commitment to change.

Ignorance is not always bliss: The pre-contemplation stage

People in this stage aren't receptive to solutions because they can't see the problem. As the saying goes, "Denial ain't just a river in Egypt." They may go on a diet because of pressure from their spouses, parents, or friends. They're typically very resistant to change and are anxious to rationalize the situation. When a discussion does begin, they change the subject or blame someone or something else. You might hear them say things like:

"I'm eating this stuff because my husband wants me to."

"It's in my genes. My whole family is fat."

"I have a low thyroid and everything I eat goes to fat."

"I can't eat better because my wife won't cook it for me."

"I can't eat better because we have to keep all these snacks in the house for the kids."

"My knees are bad and I can't exercise. Everyone knows you can't lose weight if you don't exercise."

"I can't afford to eat healthy food."

They feel the situation is hopeless. Sometimes they can't even articulate the problem. They just feel there is nothing they can do to overcome the barriers in their life.

So how does this work, anyway? The contemplation stage

People in this stage start to recognize and acknowledge that they have a problem. They begin to think about solving it. They struggle to understand the problem, to see its causes, and wonder about possible solutions. They know they want to get healthy and they know how to do it, but they aren't sure if they're ready to start. They have indefinite plans to take action within the next few months. It isn't uncommon for people in this stage to say things like:

"I really want to lose weight, and someday I'm going to do it."

"When I get through with this project, then I'm really going to start exercising and eating better."

"After I graduate from college and get out from under this stress, I'm going to take better care of myself."

When people in this stage start to transition to the preparation stage of change, their thinking is marked by two changes: They begin to think more about the future than the past; then they start to feel anticipation, anxiety, and excitement, and activity starts to occur to prepare for the change.

How do I do it? The preparation stage

People in the preparation stage are planning to take action and are making the final adjustments before they begin to change their behavior. They've purchased the walking shoes, joined the gym, stocked up on healthier food, or adjusted their schedule. However, they may not have fully resolved their ambivalence about making the change. They may still need a little convincing.

Practice makes perfect: The action stage

This is the stage where people are actually modifying their behavior and their surroundings. They take the action for which they have been preparing. They start walking. They avoid the pastry cart. They make a healthier food choice. They switch to diet colas.

This stage requires the greatest commitment of time and energy. Their changes in lifestyle become visible to others.

Creating a habit: The maintenance stage

Change never ends with the action stage. The new behavior has to become a habit. Without a strong commitment to maintenance, there will be relapse, usually to pre-contemplation or contemplation. But relapse is okay if you learn from it.

Maintenance on the Whole Foods Eating Plan is not triggered by reaching a weight or fitness goal. On this plan, maintenance simply means that you're maintaining all the good habits you've started. You aren't finished; your job is not over at this point. You must maintain these habits to maintain the benefits.

People do not move easily from one stage of change to the other. They often bounce back and forth between two stages before they move forward to the next stage. They may go through the entire process three or four times before they make it through without a setback.

Taking It Up a Notch: Moving from One Level of Commitment to the Next

As you progress through each stage, you gain important skills, learning, and insights. Whatever stage you find yourself in today, you have made significant effort and progress toward your goals.

If you're reading this book, then you're at the very least in the contemplation stage. Do the following assignments to help move you into the preparation stage.

Write out answers to the following:

 ✔ Choosing healthier foods will give me the following benefits:

 ✔ I will make the following changes to achieve a healthier diet:

Follow through on making those changes and you are now in the action stage. You're developing a self-image that is fit, and you're becoming proactive in maintaining your fitness. You see yourself in control of your health and able to rise above influences that make you less healthy.

Recording your food choices is a great way to identify good habits and a great way to identify problem areas. Keep a record of everything you eat for a week. Think about where you were, who was with you, and how you felt. Record everything. You only hurt yourself if you're not honest.

After you've recorded your food choices for the week, answer these questions:

- What days did you make the best food choices and why?
- What days did you *not* make good food choices and why?
- Was a certain time of day harder for you to make a good food choice?
- What changes can you make to ensure success in the future?

Identify your danger zones. Does sitting in the kitchen cause you to raid the pantry? Does lingering at the dinner table make you long for dessert?

Rallying Support

Don't go it alone. Find someone to be in your corner, someone who is non-judgmental and positive-minded, someone who believes in you. Carefully, and I mean *carefully*, identify one or more friends or family members who will support your efforts. Some people think the best way to get support is to announce to the world that they are "on a diet." They think that publicly making this announcement will ensure their compliance.

Be very careful if you tell people you're going on a diet. This could easily backfire on you and turn into resentment as well-meaning friends turn into food cops, policing every bite of food you put into your mouth. They may not understand your eating plan because everyone seems to have a precon-ceived idea of what you should or should not eat. (For some reason, they feel no obligation to justify their *own* food choices, of course.)

My personal recommendation is to keep your plans private except for one or two sincere supporters. You know what you can eat and not eat and how much. Just make good choices and think about something else.

After you've identified your support people, list two or more ways they can help you. Talk to them about it ahead of time and determine how they can help. Come up with a secret sign language that lets them tell you if you're about to go overboard.

When you've prepared your mind, assessed your level of commitment, gained knowledge and insight into your behavior, and created your support system, you're ready to go. *Remember:* This is a lifetime project, so don't get upset if you have an occasional slip. One bad day is no reason to quit. Forgive yourself, learn from the experience, and continue to move forward.

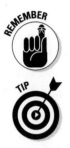

Your goals are making the right food choices and getting regular exercise. Don't set yourself up for failure by trying to achieve a predetermined number. Concentrate on developing a healthy lifestyle and then reap the benefits.

If you want to keep a record of the results of your good habits, use the following chart:

Measurement	Today	After 6 Weeks	After 12 Weeks
BMI			
Weight			
Pants size			
Waist measurement			
Bust/chest measurement			
Hip measurement			
Upper-arm measurement			
Thigh measurement			
Calf measurement			

To monitor your medical benefits, make an agreement with your physician. After your doctor does the baseline lab work that includes blood sugar, total cholesterol, HDL cholesterol, LDL cholesterol, triglycerides, blood pressure, and weight, tell him/her that you want to try lifestyle changes. Set an appointment to return in three months (or sooner if you need support) for repeat lab work to evaluate your results.

Chapter 17

Setting Yourself Up to Succeed

*I*s your home your own worst enemy? Chances are, the source of some of your greatest temptations is right in your own kitchen. The typical kitchen tends to have too many high-calorie, high-carbohydrate, and high-fat foods and too few fruits and vegetables, whole grains, lean meat, and low-fat dairy products.

You need to build an environment that supports your new healthy lifestyle. You may be tempted to give the whole place an overhaul. But your spouse and kids or other housemates may be saying, "We aren't on a diet. Don't get rid of *our* food." You don't have to toss out everyone's favorite food. Think about giving your kitchen a makeover rather than an overhaul. Tolerate some high-calorie foods in the house, but focus on eating healthier snacks. Make those healthy choices available to everyone. You may be surprised at how often other family members choose a healthy food when they have a choice.

Identifying Your Trigger Foods

Each of us has our own high-calorie foods that we just can't seem to resist. With trigger foods, a small bite just doesn't work. They're the sorts of foods that, when you start eating them, you just can't stop. If you know the food is in the house, you're constantly drawn to it as if it were a magnet. These foods are called trigger foods, because they pull the trigger on overeating and increase your hunger all day long.

You may not be aware that a certain food is a trigger food for you until you really think about it. Getting in touch with how certain foods make you feel is important. When you keep a record of your food intake as suggested in Chapter 16, record how you feel after eating a food. If a food tastes wonderful, you can't seem to get enough of it, and eating it intensifies your hunger for all foods the rest of the day, then *that* is a trigger food.

Follow these suggestions for dealing with your own trigger foods:

✔ **Exclude all trigger foods from your shopping and house.** If this is too brutal for the rest of the family, include a few of them along with healthier snack choices. Divide the trigger foods into portions and store the portions in the freezer. If you do indulge, it will already be portioned out for you.

✔ **Avoid excess hunger.** It's hard to resist anything when you're hungry, but especially trigger foods. Plan healthy between-meal snacks and never skip a meal.

✔ **Avoid letting stress contribute to overeating.** Maintain your regular meals, exercise, and sleep. Go for a walk before grabbing for the cookie jar. See Chapter 18 for tips on managing stress.

✔ **Make trigger foods less accessible.** Hide them. Store them in the highest cabinet or in the back of the freezer.

✔ **Develop some great-tasting treats from fruits, sugar-free gelatin, and sugar-free puddings.** Start with recipes in this book and then develop your own.

If you have a sweet tooth, include a lot of fruit in your diet to satisfy it. Fresh fruit at the peak of ripeness is wonderfully delicious and sweet. If fresh isn't available, try frozen or canned fruits. Mix several kinds together or try frozen bing cherries by themselves for an instant treat. Try topical fruits like mangos, and unsweetened versions of dried fruits, like raisins and dried pineapple.

Feed a craving or ignore it?

A *craving* is an intense and prolonged desire or yearning for a particular food. Most people crave foods high in sugar and fat and low in nutrients. The reasons for the craving are multiple. But, for whatever reason, you can't get the desire for a particular food out of your head and you're afraid it will lead to overeating or bingeing. So, what do you do? Give in to it and risk losing control and going overboard? Or staunchly resist it until it goes away?

If the craving is from simple boredom, you can probably divert your attention away from it. But if it's a true physiological craving, then you probably need to satisfy the craving by eating the food. Most studies indicate that deprivation does not work and may lead to a craving that results in bingeing. If you do give in to the craving, know how to control the amount you eat. Don't bring home a gallon of ice cream, a box of doughnuts, a package of cookies, or an entire pie or cake. Instead go out and buy one scoop of your favorite ice cream, or one doughnut or cookie, or one piece of cake or pie. Eat it slowly, savor each bite, and enjoy it. Then get back on track with your eating plan. One little detour off the eating plan will not upset the progress you've made. It's only when the detours become too frequent that you may be developing a problem.

Stocking the Fridge

The refrigerator is often the center of the kitchen, which in turn is the center of the home. Try to keep these staples on hand so you can whip up low-carb meals in minutes:

- Low-fat or nonfat milk, yogurt, and cheeses (with no more than 5 grams of fat per ounce)
- Fresh eggs as well as egg-substitutes or egg whites
- Tub or spray margarines with no trans-fatty acids
- Low-fat deli meats and turkey bacon
- Low-fat or nonfat salad dressing

Fruits and veggies are the original fast foods. They're packaged ready to go and you don't need a knife and fork. However, when first introducing your family to fruits and vegetables as snacks, you may need to increase their accessibility. Cut them up and have them ready to go. Store them in plastic bags or containers. Take a look at Appendix C for a ready-made grocery list full of fresh fruits and veggies.

Keep a variety of fresh fruits and veggies on hand and ready to go. Here are a few ideas to get you started:

- **Buy apples, pears, or other in-season fruits.** Let kids use the apple wedger to cut them in wedges.
- **Buy a whole watermelon, keep a bowl of watermelon chunks for an easy snack, or make up several small watermelon wedges to use as a quick side dish to a sandwich or meal.**
- **Prep your veggies as soon as you get home from the grocery store.** If you buy a head of cauliflower, cucumbers, red peppers, and so on, clean and slice them immediately. Store them in the fridge so they'll be ready for snacking when you are.

Filling the Freezer

You can buy several items to keep in the freezer to make your low-carb life easier. But make sure you save room to make meals ahead and freeze them, so you'll have healthy low-carb meals ready to go all the time.

Here's the short list of freezer must haves:

- Low-fat frozen entrees
- Individual frozen pizzas

- ✔ Frozen unbreaded fish fillets
- ✔ Lean cuts of meat and skinless poultry
- ✔ Light or sugar-free frozen yogurt or ice cream
- ✔ Sugar-free fudge bars or ice cream bars
- ✔ 100-percent fruit juice concentrates
- ✔ Frozen vegetables without sauces

Keep some blueberries, seeded cherries, or grapes in the freezer. These are great bite-sized treats and are much better for you than popsicles, frozen novelties, or even juice pops. Choose a diet lemon-lime soda, grapefruit flavored soda, or club soda to pour over a bowl of frozen fruit for a quick, delicious fruit salad.

Organizing the Cupboards and Pantry

Your pantry should have a range of foods, from dried beans and grains to ready-to-go, almost out-of-the-can foods for quick meals. However, that does not mean stock up on mac and cheese or packaged dinners. You should choose canned and jarred foods that are still processed as little as possible. Look for canned beans and tomatoes, but skip the spaghetti dinner in a box. You can get roasted red peppers or chilies in a jar, but avoid the urge to get canned soup.

Getting help with already prepped ingredients is fine, but be wary if the only prep you do is heating it in a microwave. If that's the case, the food is likely loaded with preservatives, trans fats, and chemicals your body doesn't need and won't tolerate well over the long haul.

Oils and vinegars

Look for healthy oils, like olive oil, canola oil, and peanut oil or light combination oils. These are better choices than corn oil or any kind of shortening. For details on which oils are healthy, check out Chapter 7.

Nonstick vegetable oil spray is a great addition to any pantry. You can find it in a variety of flavors, including olive oil, garlic, butter, and the like. You can buy oil misters to create your own versions of these. They're available at virtually any store that sells cookware. You can use any kind of oil you have at home. Just make sure you clean the mister occasionally instead of just refilling it, because the dregs can get rancid if you don't.

Many types of vinegar are available. Vinegars are by nature acidic. Adding an acidic food to a meal lowers the glycemic index of the meal. Keep a variety of vinegars on hand to enhance different flavors in salads. Look for different varieties (such as apple cider, balsamic, garlic, raspberry, champagne, cabernet, or zinfandel) to make your own dressings or add a quick no-carb sauce to a meal.

Marinated foods

Marinated vegetables are great as snacks and side dishes. The vinegar they contain helps lower the glycemic index of the foods you eat along with them. Most of these items can be eaten right out of the jar and make great additions to veggie trays or antipastos. Here's a list to start with:

- Sun-dried tomatoes
- Artichoke hearts
- Olives
- Capers
- Marinated vegetables (okra, beans)
- Roasted peppers
- Pickles, pickle relish
- Horseradish, Dijon, spicy, or plain mustard
- Red and white table wine (for cooking)

Canned and jarred foods

Look for these items to help you whip together easy weeknight meals.

- Canned tuna, salmon, or sardines (in water)
- Canned new white potatoes
- Canned vegetables (asparagus, carrots, green beans, mushrooms)
- Canned fruit packed in light syrup or juice
- 100-percent fruit preserves
- Canned chicken or beef bouillon
- Canned tomatoes and tomato paste
- Salsa
- Ketchup

✔ Canned or dried beans such as pinto, navy, kidney, limas, garbanzo, peas

✔ Fat-free refried beans

✔ Natural or low-sugar peanut butter

Grains

These grains are handy additions to your pantry, but remember your portion sizes:

✔ Whole-grain pasta, long-grain rice, wild rice

✔ Whole-grain flours and cornmeal

✔ Oatmeal

✔ High-fiber, no sugar, cereals

✔ Low-sugar granola or homemade granola

Check out Chapter 6 for the details on how to use your five carb choices each day.

Snacks

These snacks should be used sparingly but can help in a pinch when you need a sweet-tooth fix:

✔ Low-sugar cookies, like vanilla wafers, animal crackers, or gingersnaps

✔ Low-fat microwave popcorn

✔ Whole-grain crackers

✔ Sugar-free hot cocoa mix

✔ Sugar-free gelatin and puddings

Seasonings

Variety may be the spice of life, but what would food be without seasoning? Keep these seasonings on hand for quick additions to marinades, sauces, and one-pot meals:

✔ Salt-free seasonings

✔ Garlic and onion, fresh, minced, and powder

- ✔ Bouillon cubes or sprinkles
- ✔ Reduced-sodium soy sauce or Worcestershire sauce
- ✔ Sugar substitutes

Paying Attention to Safety

Food-borne diseases cause an estimated 76 million illnesses in the United States every year according to the Centers for Disease Control and Prevention. Don't make the mistake of only associating those illnesses with restaurants and public eating places. Even though illnesses occurring in these public places get all the press, food-related illnesses can occur right in your own home.

The cardinal rule of food safety is this: Keep hot foods hot; keep cold foods cold; and keep hands, utensils, and the kitchen clean.

- ✔ Allow sufficient cooking time for food to reach safe internal temperatures during cooking, and hold the food at a high enough temperature to prevent bacterial growth until it is served. Use a food thermometer to check temperatures.

- ✔ Go directly home upon leaving the grocery store and immediately unpack foods into the refrigerator or freezer upon your arrival.

- ✔ Wash the countertops, your hands, and utensils in warm, soapy water before and after each step of food preparation.

Allowing refrigerated foods to warm up to room temperature and allowing cooked foods to cool down to room temperature creates a temperature range conducive to bacteria growth known as the *danger zone*. Between the temperatures of 40 and 140 degrees is the prime growing temperature for bacteria. No food should be kept at that temperature for longer than two hours. The "2-40-140" rule will help you to remember the time and temperature danger zone for foods: No more than 2 hours between 40 degrees F and 140 degrees F.

Here are a few other safety tips that will help keep you and your family safe from food-borne illnesses:

- ✔ **When in doubt, throw it out.** Throw out foods with danger-signaling odors. But be aware that most food poisoning bacteria are odorless, colorless, and tasteless. Do not even *taste* a food that is suspect.

- ✔ **Use separate cutting boards for meat and poultry.** Don't use wooden cutting boards. Bacteria can live in the grooves. Sterilize cutting boards in the dishwasher. Consider buying separate colors for meat and fresh foods like veggies and bread.

✔ **Wash and disinfect sponges and towels regularly.** Launder in a bleach solution.

✔ **Avoid cross-contamination by washing all surfaces (including your hands) that have been in contact with raw meats, poultry, or eggs.**

✔ **Thaw meats or poultry in the refrigerator, not on the kitchen counter.** If you must thaw foods quickly, use cool running water or the microwave.

✔ **Do not put cooked food on a plate that was used for raw meat or poultry.** If you bring your raw steaks, chicken, or burgers to the grill on a platter, get a fresh platter for the final product.

✔ **Mix foods with utensils, not your hands.** And keep hands and utensils away from your mouth, nose, and hair.

Your refrigerator temperature should be kept at 34 to 40 degrees F. If, in your household, there is a lot of opening and shutting of the refrigerator door, keep the temperature near the lower end (34 degrees). Put food in the refrigerator quickly to prevent the growth of bacteria; don't let leftovers sit out for more than two hours (hot dishes for more than an hour). Store foods in plastic bags or covered containers. Keep meat separate from vegetables to prevent cross-contamination.

Keep your freezer at sub-freezing — 0 degrees F. Wrap food in plastic wrap and foil, or store in airtight plastic bags or sealed tubs with the date marked. Place new items in the back, and rotate existing food to the front to help use them in a timely manner. If possible, use leftovers before uncooked meat.

Nonperishable does not mean a food lasts forever; it will perish at some point. Most dry goods now have expiration dates on them. Always follow those dates, when they're available. When they're not available, here are a few guidelines:

✔ **Canned foods:** Stored properly, most unopened canned foods keep for at least one year. If the top of a can is bulging, throw it out.

✔ **Bottled foods:** Sealed, they last a few months. After they're opened, be sure to refrigerate them. Depending on the food, they can last one week to two months when opened.

✔ **Boxes and bags of food:** Sealed, they last for three months to one year; open, they last one week to three months. Store open products in airtight containers to extend their longevity and to prevent odor crossover and insect invasion.

Whole-grain flours and cornmeal may keep best in the freezer. Put the whole package in a large airtight plastic bag before freezing. When baking, take out the portion you need and let it reach room temperature before using.

Chapter 18

Falling Off the Wagon and Getting On Again

Guess what? Falling off the wagon is normal! Viewing failure as a weakness or allowing it to lower your self-esteem or self-worth doesn't make sense. And it's certainly not a reason to give up! People who are the most successful at changing a behavior go through the process three or four times before they can make it through without one slip. Slip-ups give you the opportunity to figure out where you went wrong and prevent it from happening again.

Forgiving Yourself

Okay, so you blew it. You totally lost control, threw caution to the wind, and pigged out. What are you going to do now? You're feeling low and your opinion of yourself is negative, but hold it right there! You're headed on a guilt trip, so slam on the brakes, bang a U-turn, and head the other way. You've just been granted new insight into your behavior. Use it to avoid this problem in the future.

Forgiving yourself doesn't mean accepting the behavior or making excuses for it. You need to learn from your mistake, gain more self-control, and grow in your capacity to overcome it. Not forgiving yourself makes these goals harder to reach and gives the event power over you. Release yourself from the powerful grip of your own mistakes by doing the following:

✔ **Be willing to take immediate corrective action.** If you brought tempting foods into your home, throw them out. Pick up all the trash and garbage, including your tempting foods, in your house and immediately carry it to the trash. If you pigged out at a restaurant, then go for a walk or put on an exercise tape and work out until you're hot and sweaty.

✔ **Think about how you would respond to someone who did the same thing.** Would you berate that person to the same extent that you berate yourself? Of course you wouldn't. Is your mistake worse than someone else's? Think especially of how you would respond to someone you love if you learned he was treating himself in the way you treat yourself.

✔ **Confess your mistake to a trusted partner, friend, or counselor.** Talk about it. Discuss why it happened and how bad you felt about. Develop a plan to avoid the mistake in the future.

✔ **Practice loving yourself.** You're worthy of good treatment in your body, mind, emotions, and spirit. Get past this and move on.

Analyzing the Fall

So you pulled into the drive-thru and ordered a milkshake. You feel terrible about it. Think about the conditions that led to that behavior:

✔ Were you hungry?

✔ Were you angry?

✔ Were you feeling sorry for yourself?

✔ Were you feeling you deserved it because of something good you did?

✔ Were you influenced by the restaurant sign that reminded you of a TV commercial advertising milkshakes?

✔ Was someone with you that influenced your decision?

Take time to carefully analyze what motivates you to get off track. Do you use food as comfort for depression or anger? Do you use food as a reward? Do you realize how susceptible you are to the power of suggestion? Were you unrealistic in your goal? If none of these apply and you were truly hungry, evaluate your pattern of eating. Maybe you need to eat more, earlier in the day, to prevent afternoon hunger. When you've discovered the motivation behind a poor food choice, you can plan an alternative defense.

Planning alternative defenses

When you determine what motivates you to overeat or not exercise, develop an alternate strategy. The key to any successful strategy is planning. If you don't plan how you'll deal with difficult situations, they will *happen* to you. Acting is much better than reacting, so figure out your trigger situations and make a plan to head them off. If you can't go into the employee lounge without putting money in the vending machine, don't go in the employee lounge. Bring your lunch and eat at your desk or outside. Or take a healthy snack from home when you go into the employee lounge.

You may have to try out several strategies before you find the one that works the best for you. Don't be in a hurry. If you've been struggling with making or breaking a habit, here are some ways to coax it one step at a time:

- **Set small incremental goals.** If walking a mile is just too much for you to handle, then walk for five minutes. When five minutes of walking starts to feel easy, then increase it by five more minutes and so on.

- **Set realistic expectations.** Don't go full-steam into an exercise program and become so sore you don't exercise again for a week.

- **Be your own best cheerleader.** You'd do it for someone else — why not do it for yourself? Set up a reward system. Drop a quarter in a jar each time you exercise, or try a new activity. Each time you work in all your veggies each day, drop in a dime. Use the money to buy yourself a little non-food, but decidedly decadent, treat, like a book, a magazine, or a CD.

- **Schedule time for yourself.** Set times for workouts and walks, and actually follow through with it. Plan to take some time for a relaxing lunch, to refresh your mind and renew your commitments. Or just plan time to read a chapter in a book. Whatever you like to do that's relaxing and helpful to your goal of good health (both physical and mental), make time for it.

Conquering stress

A major factor in falling off the wagon is stress. When everything is perfect (and how often does that happen?), you eat right, exercise, and have a good attitude. But a minor crisis occurs and all your best-laid plans go out the window. You give in to the power of the crisis and may not even realize it because it short-circuits your thinking processes. In fact, you aren't thinking at all; you're *reacting*.

People under stress put themselves at the bottom of their priority list. They sleep poorly (either too much or not enough), eat poorly, reduce or eliminate exercise, and drop out of social activities. If this sounds familiar, you're doing exactly the opposite of what you need to do. So accept responsibility, admit the crisis is important, and start to deal with it. Take one day at a time and be flexible. Crises, small and large, in your life are permanent. Accept the crisis, do what you can about it, and move on. Don't try to resolve all your problems at once. Break them down into manageable parts. And, most of all, continue to take care of yourself.

When you recognize that stress, not hunger, is causing you to crave food, you may be able to avoid eating as a stress reaction. Or at least you may be able to find a healthy food to satisfy the craving.

People overwhelmed by stress often reach for sugary treats to get a sugar high and escape the emotion for the moment. This never works for long because, after the initial rush, you're left feeling a little sick and sometimes depressed and guilty. If stress in your life is contributing to poor eating, work on these five areas: attitude, organization, self-control, planning, and self-care.

Attitude

Thomas Edison said, "Genius is 99 percent perspiration and 1 percent inspiration." So, chalk up genius to the right attitude. The same is true with success in any endeavor, including low-carb dieting.

- ✔ **Adjust your attitude.** Instead of looking at stressful situations as problems, focus on the solutions. Problems can become opportunities to problem-solve and practice critical thinking. And more often than not, you learn more from mistakes and obstacles than you do from an easy well-planned life.

- ✔ **Whenever possible, take charge.** Just the change in perspective of making things happen versus having things happen to you is less stressful. It may seem tough at first, but this single small thing could help you realize huge improvements in your life.

Organization

Being prepared is most of the battle. Get organized today and you'll be a step closer to winning the battle.

- ✔ **Start with organizing the regular daily chores of life.** If searching for shoes every morning makes the kids late for school, then find them the night before. Enjoy the peaceful drive to school.

- ✔ **Schedule your stress.** When you have this luxury, take advantage of it. If you have a big project due at work, it's probably not the best week to also get ready to go on vacation. If your in-laws are visiting, don't also try to organize the PTA bake sale, paint the house, and re-landscape the yard. Whatever the events in your life, ask yourself, "Do I need to do this?" and, "Do I really need to do this now?" Find what works for you.

Self-control

Self-control means knowing when to say yes and when to say no:

✔ **Just do it.** Procrastination breeds stress. If you're dreading something, then get after it and get it over with. If you're going to continue to think about doing it, just do it now, and get on with your day.

✔ **Just say, "No."** You know they can and will find somebody else. The reason you're being asked is because the person before you said, "No." Only do what you truly want to do.

Planning

Inevitable obstacles are part of life, but the more you can anticipate, the better off you are.

✔ **Set realistic goals.** Don't take on too much. Whether it's the amount of weight you're going to lose or how many errands you're going to cram into a weekend, be realistic. There is no pressure like the pressure that you put on yourself. Understand what you can actually do in a day, and do it well.

✔ **Practice it.** You can't predict every stressful event that comes up, but you can prepare for some of them. Being prepared reduces stress. If you know that you have to confront a co-worker, you can develop a plan ahead of time. Role-play with a friend to help you make it realistic. If you have to have a difficult conversation with your significant other, practice in the mirror. Find a strategy that works for you.

Self-care

You're the best person to take care of you, so start today:

✔ **Treat your body right.** Eat a healthy diet, get enough sleep, and exercise regularly. You'll reduce the stress in your life, gain energy and confidence, and be less susceptible to the side effects of stress.

✔ **Take breaks as often as you need to.** You may not be able to work in scheduled breaks throughout the day, but definitely take a few breaks, and then come back to your work refreshed. Often, you're able to complete a job much quicker if you have something fun to look forward to when you're done, like a walk around the building with a friend. Also, often a problem you're dealing with looks much different through a fresh pair of eyes, even if they're your own.

✔ **Give yourself a pep talk.** Keep telling yourself you can handle this and you will get through it. Avoid putting yourself down with negative words about your abilities.

Renewing Your Commitment

If you've tried everything but just can't seem to create the new habit, take an honest look at your motivation. Are you making the change because you really want to or because you think you should or have been told you should? You may need to go back to Chapter 16 and reassess your motivation. It may take a couple of false starts before you finally begin making progress.

If at first you don't succeed, try again. Very few people succeed at making permanent changes in their lives the first time out. Don't use failure as an excuse to quit. Everyone remembers baseball player Babe Ruth as the Home Run King. Few remember that he was also the Strike-Out King.

Learn from your mistakes, and move on. At each setback, or slipup, figure out what went wrong, and develop a strategy for heading it off the next time.

Breaking the Cycle of Failure

If you're having trouble getting from where you are to where you want to be, you may be trapped in a cycle of failure. You may be hanging on to past events and attitudes that are constantly sabotaging your efforts. For new eating habits and exercise patterns to begin, old eating habits and exercise patterns must end. Your problem may not be how to get new, innovative, healthy thoughts and behaviors into your mind, but how to get old ones out.

Success doesn't just happen. It's a constant progression of discovering what works, practicing it until it's a habit, and getting rid of what doesn't work. You can't move forward if you continue the old ways of doing things.

Here are a few ideas for getting your attitude moving in the right direction:

- **Think about what negative behaviors and attitudes are preventing you from being successful.** Are you subconsciously sabotaging your efforts because you're unwilling to give up some habits? What do you need to let go of in order to move forward?

- **Rethink and renew your commitment to yourself.** Do you really want to be a healthier person or is it someone else's idea? Are you fearful of the new person you will become?

- **Think about what else you can do to improve yourself while creating a new lifestyle.** Learn a new skill, read a book, take a class — exercise your mind as well as your body.

- **Continue striving to be healthy.** Share your experiences with someone else who is trying to become healthy. You aren't going to be the same person in the future that you are today. Start accepting and adjusting to the "new" you.

Part VI
The Part of Tens

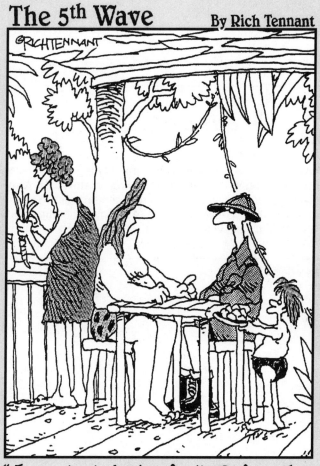

The 5th Wave — By Rich Tennant

"Jane start drying fruit. Before that we just eat cheetah. Too much fast food not good."

In this part . . .

Get ready to gauge your results. I'll show you ways to track your progress by appreciating benefits of low-carb eating other than the number on the scale. Also check out this part for answers to commonly asked questions. Finally, I've included a list of additional online resources in case you need continuing support.

Chapter 19

Ten Benefits of Low-Carb Dieting

In This Chapter
▶ Assessing your health before and after changing your eating
▶ Appreciating benefits other than weight loss

*E*ating a healthy diet and exercising have many benefits. In fact, these two activities alone are the most important things you can do to improve your health. But don't shortchange yourself when you evaluate your progress. Don't put the whole focus on the number of pounds you've lost or what you weigh. If you do, you'll be missing some of your greatest rewards. And if you give up the plan because you didn't reach the magic number on the scale, you're throwing out your greatest benefits. In this chapter, I list ten very gratifying ways to discover that you're on the right track.

Improved Glucose Control

One of the first benefits of reducing the total amount of carbohydrate (especially the refined carbohydrate foods) in your diet is usually an improvement in your blood glucose (blood sugar) level. Let the carbohydrate foods that you do choose to eat be fruits, vegetables, and whole-grain or unrefined grain foods. You'll notice fewer sugar highs and sugar lows, which create hunger.

Quality whole foods sustain you, are easier for your body to process, and are chock-full of vitamins and minerals you can't get in a pill.

Better Appetite Control

Another benefit of low-carb dieting is an improvement in your appetite. You'll have a normal hunger at mealtimes, but it will be easily satisfied by the foods on the Whole Foods Eating Plan. You'll no longer have periods of ravenous hunger. On those days when you *are* hungrier, you have a variety of Green Light foods to satisfy that hunger and still maintain your healthy eating plan. Check out Chapter 10 for planning tips and Chapter 5 for the full list of Green Light foods.

Improved Concentration

As your blood sugar becomes more stable, you'll notice that you can concentrate better. You'll no longer feel lethargic and barely able to hold your eyes open after lunch. Your focus will improve. (If you've ever found yourself reading and re-reading the same section of the newspaper, an e-mail, or a book, you know what I'm talking about.) You'll be better able to start and complete tasks quickly, with fewer interruptions.

Weight Maintenance

On the Whole Foods Eating Plan, you'll notice that you feel more comfortable in your clothes and your body feels lighter. Your weight won't increase; in fact, you'll probably lose a few pounds. Your weight loss will be slow and healthy and will continue, but remember that no weight gain is always progress. If you're on a cycle of weight gain, stopping it is extremely important to your future health.

Improved Blood Pressure

The Whole Foods Eating Plan provides low-fat dairy products, protein, calcium, potassium, magnesium, and fiber — all nutrients proven to lower your blood pressure. The Whole Foods Eating Plan allows you to rid yourself of extra water you may be retaining. This loss of excess water not only makes you feel better, it helps to lower your blood pressure. You'll notice your blood pressure is improving if you check it regularly. If you require medication to control your blood pressure, your family doctor may eventually be able to decrease the amount, or eliminate it completely.

Blood-pressure monitors in pharmacies are good places for periodic checks between doctor visits.

Improved Cholesterol

The Whole Foods Eating Plan significantly lowers your intake of saturated fat and trans fatty acids as well as lowers your overall carbohydrate intake. You're encouraged to choose monounsaturated fats and to increase your intake of fish supplying omega-3 fatty acids. These dietary changes are important in lowering your total cholesterol, LDL cholesterol, and triglyceride levels in your blood. When your physician repeats your cholesterol blood tests, you should notice an improvement in your cholesterol and triglyceride levels. Discuss this with your doctor.

Improved Sleep

Lowering the amount of carbohydrate and the amount of food that you eat in the evening will allow you to sleep better. Your body is able to fully relax because it isn't up digesting a heavy meal. Stabilizing your blood sugar and getting rid of excess water cuts down on your number of trips to the bathroom. You'll be able to sleep longer without being disturbed. You'll feel rested when you awaken in the morning because you had a good night's sleep.

And with increased physical activity, your body will become more physically tired and relaxed. You're likely to be able to more quickly settle in at night and fall asleep faster.

More Energy

You'll definitely notice that you have a lot more energy. That is partly because you'll be getting good sleep. The Whole Foods Eating Plan will provide nourishment to the cells of your body. You'll get rid of surplus water that was weighing you down. If you add exercise to the program, it will energize you. If you add strength training, you'll be burning more fuel all the time and reduce lethargic episodes.

Better Mood

When you just feel better all over, your mood improves. You'll be happier and you'll respond to people with a more positive attitude. You'll feel stronger, better, rested, and healthy. You'll be amazed at how quickly this happens, when you simply remove the stress of trying to decide how to get fit and healthy.

More Self-Confidence

It all comes together with a more confident you. Your health will improve, your appetite will be controlled, your concentration will be better, you'll be controlling your weight, you'll be sleeping better, you'll be getting more done because you have more energy, and you'll be happier and more confident. And all you'll have done was change your diet and started getting a little more exercise.

Chapter 20

Ten Frequently Asked Questions about Low-Carb Dieting

In This Chapter

▶ Finding out whether you can eat fruits and vegetables

▶ Knowing what you can eat if you're a vegetarian

▶ Getting answers to other common questions

*W*hen you start a low-carb eating plan, you're bound to have some questions. In this chapter, I specifically answer ten questions that I hear frequently from people who are following the Whole Foods Eating Plan.

Do I Count the Carbohydrate in Fruits and Vegetables?

Fruits and vegetables contain carbohydrate, but this is good carbohydrate that your body thrives on. Don't count the carbohydrate in fruits (except bananas). And don't count the carbohydrate in vegetables if they're non-starchy. Starchy fruits and vegetables — such as bananas, potatoes, corn, dried beans (pinto, garbanzo, navy, limas, butterbeans), English peas, and black-eyed peas — all count in your carbohydrate allowance.

Can I Use Dried Beans and Peas as Meat Substitutes?

Dried beans and peas are a good source of protein and are often referred to as a substitute for meat, which they can be. However, they also contain carbohydrate — but this carb is good carb. If your meal includes meat, count the dried beans and peas as a carbohydrate. If your meal doesn't include meat, count about 1 to 1½ cups of the beans as a portion of meat and not as a carb — this serving of beans would be free as a lean protein. Count any additional beans or peas beyond this amount as a carb.

How Do I Follow a Lower-Carbohydrate Diet If I'm a Vegetarian?

If you're a vegetarian, lower your intake of processed carbs and reduce your portion sizes of the other carbohydrates. The important thing to remember is that you want the carbohydrates you eat to be good ones. Here's a list of the different types of vegetarian diets and how to make adjustments to the Whole Foods Eating Plan if you are trying to lose weight:

✓ **Strict vegetarian or vegan:** If you're practicing a vegan lifestyle, ensure that you're getting enough soy products to maintain adequate calcium intake. Count soymilk as dairy and count all legumes as lean proteins. You may want to consider taking a vitamin B_{12} supplement as well.

✓ **Lacto vegetarian:** A lacto vegetarian consumes milk and other dairy products in addition to plant foods. On the Whole Foods Eating Plan, you'll get your two servings of dairy and then add legumes and/or soy products to ensure you get enough protein.

✓ **Lacto-ovo vegetarian:** To qualify for this status, you'll eat eggs as well as milk and other dairy products in addition to plant foods. Keep your dairy servings to two or three per day, your egg servings to one per day, and bump up your intake of legumes and soy products.

✓ **Pescovegetarian:** If you eat no red meats but consume fish as well as plant foods, but no dairy, be sure to include unfried seafood in your diet every day. Legumes and soy products should probably make an appearance in your diet, especially to ensure you get enough calcium.

✓ **Pollovegetarian:** If you eat no red meats or dairy but do eat poultry and plant foods, you shouldn't have much trouble with the diet. Count your poultry as your lean protein, and add soy products or a calcium supplement to ensure that you're getting adequate calcium each day.

What If I Just Eat the Green Light Foods and Nothing Else?

If you eat just the Green Light foods, you won't get enough carbohydrate, plus you'll be omitting milk, monounsaturated fats, and whole grains and starchy vegetables. If you eat only the Green Light foods, you're following a *very*-low-carbohydrate diet and you could end up in *ketosis* (the process of burning fat for fuel). Ketosis for extended periods of time can lead to problems in some people.

Do I Need to Take a Vitamin/Mineral Supplement?

If you follow the Whole Foods Eating Plan exactly as recommended, you may not need a vitamin/mineral supplement. You should be able to get all your nutrients from the food in your diet. However, if you have a chronic illness like diabetes or high blood pressure or heart disease, you may want to add some supplements to your diet to prevent worsening of the disease. Also, if you're at risk for osteoporosis, you may want to start taking a calcium supplement to lessen the disease's impact. Certain age groups need more of some vitamins or minerals. See Chapter 14 for more information.

How Much Weight Can I Expect to Lose?

Weight loss varies among individuals. The more overweight or obese you are, the greater your initial weight loss will be. The initial weight loss is usually the greatest weight loss because you're losing water. You won't continue to lose at this same rate for the duration of the diet. After a few weeks on the diet, your weight loss will level off to 1 to 2 pounds per week. The closer you get to your desirable weight, the slower the weight loss.

Don't focus on a number on a scale to evaluate your progress. Concentrate on eating a healthy, satisfying diet and let the weight loss just be a side effect.

Is a Low-Carb Diet Safe for Kids?

A very-low-carb diet is totally inappropriate for children. The Whole Foods Eating Plan was not designed for kids. Children and teenagers need the nutrients provided by milk and starchy foods. At a minimum, children over the age of 2 years need four 8-ounce servings of low-fat or skim milk per day. Carbohydrate foods are necessary for growth and energy. Five servings a day is too few for active children. Six to eleven servings of breads, cereals, and starchy vegetables are more appropriate. The concept of free lean protein, fruits, and vegetables still applies. If your child's diet consists of a lot of soft drinks, cookies, candy, or other refined carbohydrate or fast food, reducing the intake of those foods is a good idea.

What Can I Keep in the House for When I'm in a Hurry?

A quick change in plans can easily cause you to grab fast food. Plan for these events because they will happen — it's part of life. If you think a situation through and plan what you will do before it happens, you've won the battle. Plan to have quick meals in the freezer or a meal you can whip up from canned goods in the pantry. Many good-quality frozen dinners or entree items are suitable for a lower-carb eating plan. Keep a few of those in the freezer. You can zap one in the microwave and prepare a side salad, have a piece of fruit, and add a glass of skim milk faster than you can go pick something up. You'll feel better physically and mentally by doing this. And you'll be better prepared to deal with the crisis.

How Do I Control Cravings?

In the early stages of a low-carb diet, you may crave carbs. That's why planning some between-meal snacks is smart. Try a protein food combined with a fruit or vegetable (for example, mozzarella string cheese and grapes or cottage cheese and tomatoes). If you notice the craving occurs about the same time every day, intervene with a snack 30 minutes earlier. Cravings can occur from erratic eating patterns, skipped meals, and diets high in refined carbohydrate. Overall, when you adapt to a lower-carbohydrate eating plan, you will have better appetite control and fewer cravings.

If you just can't resist an urge for something sweet, then don't bake a cake or bring home a gallon of ice cream. Purchase a single portion of the food. Eat it slowly. Savor the taste. And then get back on your plan. You may save two or three of your carbohydrate choices to spend that way on occasion. Just compensate for the splurge by eating wisely at your other meals. If you just have a sweet tooth, satisfy it with the natural sweetness of fruit.

What Do I Do When I Just Can't Keep to the Five Carbohydrate Choices per Day?

When you're in a situation that prevents following the five carb choices, always practice portion control. Try as much as possible to concentrate on foods that meet your eating plan, but if you're in a situation that just won't work, eat smaller portions. This will get you through the meal or situation. You can always balance the extra carbohydrate intake by just choosing lean protein, fruits, and vegetables at the next meal. Don't skip the meal just because the food choices aren't right. Meal skipping can do more harm in the long run.

Chapter 21

Ten Sources of Help on the Web

- -

In This Chapter

▶ Locating health resources online

▶ Finding a registered dietitian in your area

▶ Determining which online information is accurate

- -

The World Wide Web is the fastest source of information on any topic. The important thing to keep in mind, however, is that anyone can post information on the Web, accurate or not. You have to be a discerning user of the information you have.

In this chapter, I list ten Web sites that I know to be sources of reliable information — I use them myself. If you aren't familiar with using the Web, sometimes referred to as the Internet, visit your local public library. The staff will be happy to show you how to access any of the sites I list here. Pick out a couple that appeal to you and enjoy an hour or two of surfing the Net.

The American Dietetic Association

The American Dietetic Association (ADA) is my professional organization and the nation's largest organization of food and nutrition professionals. The mission of the ADA is to serve the public by promoting nutrition, health, and well-being. One way they do this is by providing a wealth of information for consumers and the media on their Web site (www.eatright.org). Just click on the Food and Nutrition Information bar to begin accessing the information. If you want to find the services of a Registered Dietitian (RD), you can use the Find a Nutrition Professional feature on the ADA's Web site. The site contains a Tip of the Day and a Monthly Feature of timely nutrition information. Other consumer features are the Nutrition Fact Sheets, FAQs, and the Good Nutrition Reading List. This is the best site to begin with in finding quick and accurate information on a multitude of nutrition topics.

If you want more information, you can also write the American Dietetic Association at 120 South Riverside Plaza, Suite 2000, Chicago, IL 60606-6995, or call them at 800-877-1600.

The American Medical Association

The American Medical Association (AMA) is the organization of America's physicians. The AMA sets standards for medical education, practice, and ethics. The AMA Web site (www.ama-assn.org) features a consumer health area providing patients with reliable healthcare information from introductory to more advanced levels. It contains Medem's award-winning *Medical Library* representing a full range of patient education information.

Here's a quick list of features you might find interesting:

- ✔ Learning Centers with articles conveniently organized around popular topics
- ✔ Medical News sections that highlight the latest information from Medem's medical societies
- ✔ *Smart Parents' Health Source,* a free children's health e-newsletter

Tufts University Nutrition Navigator

There is so much information on the Tufts Nutrition Navigator Web site (www.navigator.tufts.edu) that if you're new to the Internet there's no reason to go anywhere else for a while. This site contains a huge volume of nutrition information that has already been evaluated for you. The Web sites are reviewed by nutritionists from Tufts University for accuracy and then given a rating. You can trust the information you find here. This site not only helps you find information quickly that is best suited to your needs, it's fun to use and has online interactive quizzes to test your knowledge.

WebMD

WebMD (www.webmd.com) provides valuable health information on a variety of topics, not just nutrition. It provides helpful tools for managing your health. The content is timely and credible. This is the site to go to if you have a new diagnosis or a friend or family member with a health problem that you don't understand. The information is very comprehensive.

USDA Food and Nutrition Center

The Food and Nutrition Information Center (FNIC) is part of the U.S. Department of Agriculture's 1971 mission to collect and disseminate information about food and human nutrition to the general public. The Web site (`www.nal.usda.gov/fnic`) contains information on food safety, dietary guidelines, reports and studies, and online resources.

The Consumer Corner feature contains information about the food and nutrition topics the public most frequently asks about. The information on this site is extremely reliable; it's prepared by federal health agencies and food and nutrition specialists from Cooperative Extension Departments across the Nation.

Healthy Living — Nutrition

Healthy Living — Nutrition (`www.bbc.co.uk/health/nutrition`) is a health and nutrition consumer education Web site sponsored by the British Broadcasting Company (BBC). The site includes basic nutrition advice, such as how to get the most nutrition for your food dollar/pound/euro, how to choose wisely when ordering from a restaurant menu, and what to consider when planning kids' meals. Some of the pages link to other BBC-authored articles, which is a nice feature if you're looking for more information on a certain topic. The Cool Tools section includes a BMI calculator, a healthy eating quiz, and a feature that lets you calculate your life expectancy based on age, personal habits, and family health history. Check out Chapter 4 for other tips on assessing your own family medical history.

ConsumerLab.com

Consumer Lab (`www.consumerlab.com`) is the Web site to visit to check out health and nutritional products such as vitamins, minerals, herbal products, and sports and energy supplements. Consumer Lab conducts independent tests to evaluate a product's quality, potency, usability by the body, and consistency. Products meeting Consumer Lab standards are allowed to carry a CL Seal of Approval. You can also find recalls and warnings about products currently on the market and information about products making false claims.

National Heart, Blood, and Lung Institute

The National Heart, Blood, and Lung Institute (NHLBI) Health Information Center (`www.nhlbi.nih.gov`) develops and maintains information on numerous topics to respond to inquiries on specific diseases related to the heart, lungs, and blood. The NHLBI Health Information Center supports and disseminates materials for the National High Blood Pressure Education Program, the

National Cholesterol Education Program, the National Heart Attack Alert Program, the National Asthma Education and Prevention Program, the NHLBI Obesity Education Initiative, and the National Center for Sleep Disorders Research, all of which are coordinated by the NHLBI.

Public and patient education materials are available on numerous topics including cholesterol, high blood pressure, asthma, heart disease, exercise, obesity, sleep disorders, and stroke.

Quackwatch

The main purpose of Quackwatch (www.quackwatch.org) is to combat fraud, myths, fads, and fallacies in the health field. This is a hard-hitting site developed by Stephen Barrett, MD. Not only is quackery-related information targeted, but quack individuals are named. You'll find information here that you won't find anywhere else. One of the goals of the site is to improve the quality of information on the Internet. Just reviewing this site will show you how to recognize information that may be coming from dubious sources.

The National Weight Control Registry

I like the National Weight Control Registry (www.nwcr.ws) because it is helping to dispel the myth that everyone who loses weight will eventually gain it back. The site was developed by Rena Wing, PhD, of Brown University and the University of Pittsburg, and by James Hill, PhD, of the University of Colorado. These researchers have identified almost 3,000 people who have lost at least 30 pounds of weight and have kept it off for one year or longer. New people who meet the qualifications are continually being added to the Registry. If you are at least 18 years old, you could be one of the new recruits.

The National Weight Control Registry publishes articles describing the eating and exercise habits and behavioral strategies used by people to be successful in weight loss and weight maintenance. An interesting feature is Success Stories, which are the inspirational weight-loss stories of some of the Registry members. Check out this site to find out what successful "losers" do.

Part VII
Appendixes

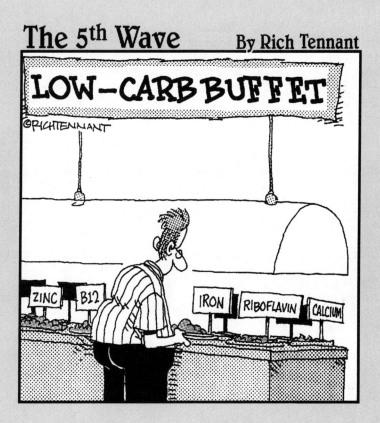

The 5th Wave   By Rich Tennant

©RICHTENNANT

LOW-CARB BUFFET

ZINC   B12   IRON   RIBOFLAVIN   CALCIUM

In this part . . .

1 include a few of my favorite tools for low-carb dieting, including the glycemic index of common foods, for your reference as you plan your meals throughout your low-carb lifestyle. Take a look at the Body Mass Index (BMI) to gauge your progress as you continue on your path to good health. Check out the appropriate levels of vitamins and minerals so you'll know the right amount to take. I also include a great shopping list to help your low-carb food selection. Enjoy!

Appendix A

The Body Mass Index

*T*he Body Mass Index (BMI) is a tool used by healthcare professionals and nutritionists to assess your general risk of health problems associated with your body size. The BMI correlates with body fat. As your BMI increases, your risk of experiencing obesity-related health problems — such as type-2 diabetes, heart disease, high blood pressure, stroke, osteoarthritis, and some cancers — increases. You can use the BMI to begin assessing your own risks and to make some healthy changes in your lifestyle.

To assess your own BMI, find your height in the far left-hand column of Table A-1. Point to it. Slowly move your finger to the right and stop when you come to the number closest to your current weight. Trace the column all the way up to the top row of bold numbers, ranging from 19 to 40. The number that's in the same column as your weight is your BMI. Now take your BMI and compare it to Table A-2.

Here's an example: Let's say Chris is 5'6" and weighs 173 pounds. Her BMI is 28. Chris is overweight and has a low degree of developing health problems based just on her weight. The BMI is only one of many factors used to predict risk for disease. She may have increased risk of health problems due to other conditions such as high blood pressure or high blood sugar. In this example, dropping her BMI by a little over 3 points would lower Chris's obesity-related health risk dramatically, by moving her from the overweight class to the normal class. She could improve her BMI, in this case, by a little over 3 points by losing 20 pounds.

But regardless of your current BMI, if you drop it by only 2 points, you'll improve your health. A weight loss of 10 percent of your current weight will significantly help to lower your risk of disease.

Table A-1   **Body Mass Index (BMI)**

Height	19	20	21	22	23	24	25	26	27	28	29	30	31	32	33	34	35	36	37	38	39	40
4'10"	91	96	100	105	110	115	119	124	129	134	138	143	148	153	158	162	167	172	177	181	186	191
4'11"	94	99	104	109	114	119	124	128	133	138	143	148	153	158	163	168	178	179	188	193	198	204
5'	97	102	107	112	118	123	128	133	138	143	148	153	158	163	168	174	179	184	189	194	199	204
5'1"	100	106	111	116	122	127	132	137	143	148	153	158	164	169	174	180	185	190	195	201	206	211
5'2"	104	109	115	120	126	131	136	142	147	153	158	164	169	174	180	186	191	196	202	207	213	218
5'3"	107	113	118	124	130	135	141	146	152	158	163	169	175	180	186	191	197	203	208	214	220	225
5'4"	110	116	122	128	134	140	145	151	157	163	169	174	180	186	192	197	204	209	215	221	227	232
5'5"	114	120	126	132	138	144	150	156	162	168	174	180	186	192	198	204	210	216	222	228	234	240
5'6"	118	124	130	136	142	148	155	161	167	173	179	186	192	198	204	210	216	223	229	235	241	247
5'7"	121	127	134	140	146	153	159	166	172	178	185	191	198	204	211	217	223	230	236	242	249	255
5'8"	125	131	138	144	151	158	164	171	177	184	190	197	203	210	216	223	230	236	243	249	256	262
5'9"	128	135	142	149	155	162	169	176	182	189	196	203	209	216	223	230	236	243	250	257	263	270
5'10"	132	139	146	153	160	167	174	181	188	195	202	209	216	222	229	236	243	250	257	264	271	278
5'11"	136	143	150	157	165	172	179	186	193	200	208	215	222	229	236	243	250	257	265	272	279	286
6'	140	147	154	162	169	177	184	191	199	206	213	221	228	235	242	250	258	265	272	279	287	294
6'1"	144	151	159	166	174	182	189	197	204	212	219	227	235	242	250	257	265	272	280	268	295	302
6'2"	148	155	163	171	179	186	194	202	210	218	225	233	241	249	256	264	272	280	287	295	303	311
6'3"	152	160	168	176	184	192	200	208	216	224	232	240	248	256	264	272	279	287	295	303	311	319
6'4"	156	164	172	180	189	197	205	213	221	230	238	246	254	263	271	279	287	295	304	312	320	328

Source: National Heart, Lung, and Blood Institute (NHLBI)

Table A-2   Classification of Overweight and Obesity Based on BMI

BMI	Obesity Class	Degree of Medical Risk
Less than 19	Underweight	Needs further assessment*
19.0 to 24.9	Normal	None
25 to 29.9	Overweight	Low
30 to 34.9	Obesity I	Moderate
35 to 39.9	Obesity II	High
40 or greater	Extreme Obesity III	Very high

* Body weights under a BMI of 19 need individualized assessment. Very lean people with low BMIs are a mix of those with illnesses associated with weight loss like cancer, emphysema, or heart disease, and a small group of physically active people or people who inherit small body size.

BMI is calculated with the same formula for children and adults, but the results are interpreted differently. For people ages 2 to 20 years, BMI is plotted on a growth chart specific for their age and gender. Be sure to check with your family doctor in evaluating your child's weight.

Appendix B

The Glycemic Index and Glycemic Load of Foods

• •

*C*arbohydrate provides energy in the form of glucose to the body. Carbohydrate foods are foods rich in carbohydrate usually in the form of sugar or starch. These foods can be digested or converted into glucose for the body. Fruits, vegetables, beans, corn, potatoes, bread, cake, cookies, sugar, and rice are easily recognized as carbohydrate foods.

Traditionally, carbohydrate foods have been divided into two categories based on their chemical structure — simple and complex. It was generally accepted that the effect on blood sugar levels was tied to a carbohydrate's chemical structure. Simple carbohydrate foods such as orange juice and apple juice were thought to raise blood sugar levels quickly, while complex carbohydrate foods such as bread and potatoes were thought to raise blood sugar levels more slowly.

This thinking was fully accepted and unchallenged until 1981 when researchers David Jenkins and Thomas Wolever of the University of Toronto published a study suggesting glycemic index be used to classify carbohydrate foods rather than the two-category system of simple and complex. This revolutionized current thinking because complex carbohydrates such as bread and potatoes were found to be digested quickly with a quick rise in blood sugar, while simple carbohydrate foods like orange juice and apple juice were digested more slowly with a moderate rise in blood sugar levels. As enlightening as this research is, the issue continues to be controversial in the United States.

In this appendix, I tell you what you need to know about the glycemic index and glycemic load, clearing up some of the confusion.

What Is the Glycemic Index?

The glycemic index (GI) describes the type of carbohydrate in a food and its ability to raise your blood sugar. The glycemic index is a value that tells how fast a particular food will raise your blood sugar. A high glycemic index value is 70 or more; moderate is in the 40 to 69 range; and low is 39 or less.

The *glycemic index value* is based on 50 grams of carbohydrate in the food without consideration for how much of the food it takes to supply 50 grams of carbohydrate. For example, a slice of bread has a high glycemic index value of 73. It takes slightly over 3 slices of bread to supply 50 grams of carbohydrate. On the other hand, a carrot has a high glycemic index value of 92, but it takes about a dozen raw carrots to give you 50 grams of carbohydrate.

What Is the Glycemic Load?

The glycemic load (GL) is a value of how much a standard *serving* of a food will raise your blood sugar. The lower the glycemic load value, the less a *serving* will spike your blood sugar. A high glycemic load value is 20 or more; moderate is in the 11 to 19 range; and low is 10 or less. When you're choosing which foods to eat, you want to shoot for foods with a lower glycemic load.

The glycemic load value is calculated by multiplying the amount of carbohydrate in a serving by the glycemic index of the food divided by 100. For example, an apple has a GI of 38, which puts it in the low category for GI. A serving of an apple (1 medium apple) contains 15 grams of carbohydrate. So $38 \times 15 = 570$, and $570 \div 100 = 5.7$ (rounded to 6). So, the apple has a low glycemic index and a low glycemic load.

On the other hand, a piece of chocolate cake with chocolate frosting also has a GI of 38, which puts it in the low category for GI. So, you might think, "Hey, chocolate cake is low glycemic and I can eat a lot of it." But an average 4-ounce serving of chocolate cake with frosting contains 52 grams of carbohydrate. So, $38 \times 52 = 1,976$, and $1,976 \div$ by $100 = 19.76$ (rounded to 20). This puts chocolate cake in the high glycemic load category. This should tell you to be careful about your portion size of chocolate cake and not to eat it too frequently. (Eat the apple instead.)

Remember those carrots with a GI of 92 (really high). Well, there are only 5 grams of carbohydrate in a 4-ounce serving, making the glycemic load 4.6 (rounded to 5, which is really low).

This helps explain why the glycemic load value is better than the glycemic index value in evaluating the foods you eat.

What Alters the Glycemic Value of a Food?

The glycemic value of a food is affected by how the carbohydrate in the food is changed during cooking, how much processing the carbohydrate in the food has undergone, and the amount of fiber in the food. Adding a small amount of fat or oil to a food (such as soft margarine of olive oil) or a little acid (such as lemon juice or vinegar) will lower the glycemic effect of the food.

Why Are Glycemic Values Important?

Food plans that incorporate low-glycemic foods over high-glycemic foods are not based on starvation and deprivation. These plans consider the *kind* of carbohydrate you eat, not the amount. Low-glycemic foods do not stimulate food cravings, do not elevate blood sugar or insulin, and do not promote fat storage.

Eating *only* low-glycemic foods isn't necessary. You can eat high-glycemic foods occasionally, as long as you keep your intake of low-glycemic foods greater than your intake of high-glycemic foods. Also watch your portion sizes of higher-glycemic foods. Coca-Cola has a GI of 63 and a GL of 16. This may make you think that Coke has a moderate GI and a moderate GL. But the GL is calculated on an 8-ounce serving. That 12-ounce can of Coke has a GL of 25 and a 20-ounce bottle has a GL of 38! (Don't even ask what the GL of a 32-ounce Coke at your favorite fast-food restaurant is.)

Where Can I Get More Information?

You can find more information on glycemic index and glycemic load as well as an online database of the GI and GL of foods at www.glycemicindex.com. This Web site is from the University of Sydney, Australia, where considerable research is being conducted on the glycemic value of foods. In addition to the database, the site provides the latest information on new GI data and research.

Appendix C

Sample Grocery List

....

In this appendix, I provide you with a sample grocery list, which you can photocopy and use again and again as you go to the store. Check out Chapters 5, 6, 7, and 8 for the full details and definitions of Green Light and Yellow Light foods.

Green Light Fruits

Fresh fruits

_____ Apples

_____ Apricots

_____ Blackberries

_____ Blueberries

_____ Cantaloupe

_____ Cherries, sweet

_____ Figs

_____ Grapefruit

_____ Grapes

_____ Honeydew melon

_____ Kiwi

_____ Lemon

_____ Lime

_____ Mango

_____ Nectarine

_____ Orange

_____ Papaya

_____ Peach

_____ Pear

_____ Pineapple

_____ Plums

_____ Raspberries

_____ Strawberries

_____ Tangerines

_____ Watermelon

Dried/canned fruits

_____ Apples, dried

_____ Applesauce, unsweetened

_____ Apricots, dried

_____ Cherries, sweet, canned, light

_____ Dates

_____ Figs, dried

_____ Fruit cocktail, light

_____ Grapefruit sections, canned, light

_____ Mandarin oranges, canned, light

_____ Peaches, canned, light

_____ Pears, canned, light

_____ Pineapple, canned, chunks, in own juice

_____ Pineapple, canned, crushed, in own juice

_____ Plums, canned, light

_____ Prunes, dried

_____ Raisins

Fruit juices

_____ Apple juice/cider

_____ Cranberry juice cocktail, reduced-calorie

_____ Fruit juice blends, 100-percent juice

_____ Grape juice

_____ Grapefruit juice

_____ Orange juice

_____ Pineapple juice

_____ Prune juice

Other fruits

_____

_____

_____

Green Light Vegetables

Fresh veggies

_____ Artichoke

_____ Asparagus

_____ Bean sprouts

_____ Beans (green, wax, Italian)

_____ Beets

_____ Broccoli

_____ Brussels sprouts

_____ Cabbage

_____ Carrots

_____ Cauliflower

_____ Celery

_____ Cucumber

_____ Eggplant

_____ Green onions or scallions

_____ Greens (collard, kale, mustard, turnip)

_____ Kohlrabi

_____ Leeks

_____ Mushrooms

_____ Okra

_____ Onions

_____ Peppers, bell, any color

_____ Peppers, hot, any variety

_____ Radishes

_____ Salad greens (endive, escarole, lettuce, romaine, spinach)

_____ Snow peas

_____ Spinach

_____ Squash, summer

_____ Tomatoes

_____ Turnips

_____ Watercress

_____ Zucchini

Canned veggies

_____ Artichoke hearts

_____ Asparagus

_____ Beans (green, wax, Italian)

_____ Beets

_____ Carrots

_____ Mushrooms

_____ Salsa or picante sauce

_____ Sauerkraut

_____ Spinach

_____ Tomato sauce

_____ Tomato/vegetable juice

_____ Tomatoes

_____ Water chestnuts

Other vegetables

_____

_____

_____

Green Light Proteins

Beef

_____ Corned beef

_____ Flank steak

_____ Ground beef, lean

_____ Ground beef, regular

_____ Prime rib

_____ Roast (rib, chuck, rump)

_____ Round

_____ Short ribs

_____ Sirloin

_____ Steak (T-bone, porterhouse)

_____ Tenderloin

Pork

_____ Boston butt

_____ Canadian bacon

_____ Center loin chop

_____ Cutlet, unbreaded

_____ Ham, canned

_____ Ham, cured

_____ Ham, deli-style

_____ Ham, fresh

_____ Tenderloin

Lamb

_____ Chop

_____ Leg

_____ Roast

Eggs

_____ Eggs, white

_____ Eggs, brown

Cheese

_____ Cheddar, reduced-fat

_____ Colby, reduced-fat

_____ Cottage cheese

_____ Feta

_____ Mozzarella

_____ Parmesan

_____ Ricotta

Fish

_____ Catfish

_____ Cod

_____ Flounder

_____ Grouper

_____ Haddock

_____ Halibut

_____ Herring

_____ Mahimahi

_____ Mackerel

_____ Pompano

_____ Orange roughy

_____ Salmon

_____ Scrod

_____ Snapper

_____ Sole

_____ Swordfish

_____ Trout

_____ Tuna, ahi

_____ Tuna, albacore

_____ Tuna, yellowfin

Poultry

_____ Chicken, breast, bone-in

_____ Chicken, breast, boneless

_____ Chicken, fryer, whole

_____ Chicken, ground

_____ Chicken, legs

_____ Chicken, pieces, pick of chick

_____ Chicken, stuffer, whole

_____ Chicken, tenders

_____ Chicken, thighs, boneless

_____ Chicken, wings

_____ Cornish hen

_____ Duck

_____ Goose

_____ Turkey, breast

_____ Turkey, legs

_____ Turkey, ground

_____ Turkey, whole

Veal

_____ Chop

_____ Cutlet, unbreaded

_____ Roast

Game

_____ Alligator

_____ Buffalo

_____ Emu

_____ Ostrich

_____ Rabbit

_____ Venison

Canned proteins

_____ Anchovies

_____ Chicken, canned

_____ Crab meat

_____ Ham, canned

_____ Salmon

_____ Sardines

_____ Shrimp

_____ Tuna, canned

Shellfish and mollusks

_____ Clams

_____ Crab

_____ Crawfish

_____ Lobster

_____ Mussels

_____ Oysters

_____ Scallops

_____ Shrimp

Other proteins

_____

_____

_____

Dairy Foods

Choose 2 to 3 servings from this list and don't forget to look at the cheese part of the Green Light protein list for extra calcium.

_____ Buttermilk

_____ Milk, lactose-free, low-fat

_____ Milk, 1%

_____ Milk, skim

_____ Yogurt, fruited, fat-free

_____ Yogurt, fruited, low-fat

_____ Yogurt, plain, fat-free

_____ Yogurt, plain, low-fat

Yellow Light Carbs

Remember, you get 5 carbohydrate choices each day from this list. Look for total carbohydrate on the food label to be about 15 grams per serving for one carbohydrate choice. You can subtract the fiber from the total carbohydrate value.

Breads

_____ Bagel

_____ Bread, reduced-calorie

_____ Bread, white

_____ Bread, whole-wheat

_____ Bread, pumpernickel

_____ Bread, rye

_____ Breadsticks, crisp

_____ English muffin

_____ Hamburger buns

_____ Hot dog buns

_____ Pita

_____ Raisin bread, unfrosted

_____ Roll, plain

_____ Tortilla, corn

_____ Tortilla, flour

_____ Waffle, reduced-fat

Vegetables and fruits

_____ Banana

_____ Corn

_____ Mixed vegetables

_____ Peas

_____ Plantain

_____ Popcorn

_____ Potato

_____ Squash, acorn or butternut

_____ Sweet potato

Legumes

_____	Black beans	_____	Lima beans
_____	Black-eyed peas	_____	Peanuts
_____	Garbanzo beans	_____	Pinto beans
_____	Kidney beans	_____	White beans
_____	Lentils		

Grains and cereals

_____	Bran cereals	_____	Kasha
_____	Bulgur	_____	Millet
_____	Cereal, cooked	_____	Muesli
_____	Cereal, sugar-frosted	_____	Oats
_____	Cereal, unsweetened	_____	Pasta
_____	Cornmeal, dry	_____	Puffed cereal
_____	Couscous	_____	Quinoa
_____	Flour, dry	_____	Rice, brown
_____	Granola, low-fat	_____	Rice, white
_____	Grape-Nuts	_____	Shredded Wheat
_____	Grits	_____	Wheat germ

Soy products

_____	Edamame (green soybeans)	_____	Tempeh
_____	Miso	_____	Tofu, extra firm
_____	Soy milk	_____	Tofu, silken
_____	Soy nuts		

Other Elements of a Low-Carb Lifestyle

_____	Broth, beef	_____	Brown Sugar sweetener
_____	Broth, chicken	_____	Cake mix, sugar-free
_____	Broth, vegetable	_____	Cooking spray, nonfat

_____ Crystal Light

_____ Gelatin, sugar-free

_____ Mayonnaise, reduced-fat

_____ NutraSweet

_____ Pudding, sugar-free, fat-free

_____ Salad dressing, reduced-fat

_____ Sour cream, reduced-fat

_____ Splenda

Dietary Reference Intakes

• •

*Y*ou may be familiar with Recommended Dietary Allowances (RDAs), but you may not have heard of Dietary Reference Intakes (DRIs). DRIs were established in 1997 by the Food and Nutrition Board, and they're based on several factors, including the RDAs. Put simply, the RDAs are a part of the DRIs, but they aren't the whole story.

The Dietary Reference Intakes don't just talk about how much of the various vitamins and minerals you should have. It also addresses issues such as exercise, sugar consumption, and how many of your calories should come from protein versus carbohydrates. In this appendix, I sort through the report and give you only the information you need.

Vitamins and Minerals

The DRIs represent a shift in focus from preventing vitamin and mineral deficiency to decreasing the risk of chronic disease. The levels recommended in the DRIs may reduce your risk of cardiovascular disease, osteoporosis, certain cancers, and other diet-related diseases.

If you take vitamin and mineral supplements, pay particular attention to the new RDAs as a goal for your average daily intake from food and supplements and the ULs (Tolerable Upper Intake Level) as an indicator of the highest amount you can take safely.

Table D-1 lists the new RDAs that are part of the DRIs. Table D-2 lists the ULs (the maximum you can take safely).

Table D-1	New RDAs for Men and Women Ages 19 to 50	
Vitamin or Mineral	*Men*	*Women*
Vitamin A (IU/d)	2333 IU	3000 IU
Vitamin C (mg/d)	75	90
Vitamin D (IU)	200 IU	200 IU
Vitamin E (IU/d)	15 IU	15 IU
Vitamin K (mcg/d)	90	120
Thiamin (mg/d)	1.1	1.2
Riboflavin (mg/d)	1.1	1.3
Niacin (mg/d)	14	16
B6 (mg/d)	1.3	1.3
Folate (mcg/d)	400	400
B12 (mcg/d)	2.4	2.4
Calcium (mg/d)	1,000	1,000
Phosphorus (mg/d)	700	700
Magnesium (mg/d)	420	320
Iron (mg/d)	18	8
Zinc (mg/d)	8	11
Selenium (mcg/d)	55	55

Table D-2	ULs for Men and Women Ages 19 to 70
Vitamin or Mineral	*Upper Limit*
Vitamin A (IU/d)	10,000 IU
Vitamin C (mg/d)	2,000
Vitamin D (IU)	2,000 IU
Vitamin E (IU)	1,000 IU synthetic; 1,500 IU natural
Niacin (mg/d)	35
B6 (mg/d)	100
Folate (mcg/d)	1,000

Vitamin or Mineral	Upper Limit
Calcium (mg/d)	2,500
Phosphorus (mg/d)	4,000
Magnesium (mg/d)	350 (non-food)
Iron (mg/d)	45
Zinc (mg/d)	40
Selenium (mcg/d)	400 (mcg/d)

Carbohydrate, Protein, and Fat

In 2002, a DRI report addressed the question of how much carbohydrate, fat, and protein you need to consume on a daily basis to ensure good health. The ranges are new and are geared toward achieving a nutritionally adequate diet while minimizing your risk of developing chronic disease.

Here are the recommended percentages:

- ✔ **Carbohydrate:** 45 to 65 percent of calories
- ✔ **Fat:** 20 to 35 percent of calories
- ✔ **Protein:** 10 to 35 percent of calories

An amount of 130 grams of total carbohydrate was set as a minimum amount for both children and adults. This newly set DRI is based on the amount of carbs your body needs in order to provide enough glucose for the brain to function and to prevent loss of lean body mass. Very-low-carbohydrate diets of 20 to 30 grams of total carbohydrate fall far short of this goal. (The Whole Foods Eating Plan outlined in this book falls well within the new DRI.)

Sugar

According to the DRI report, no more than 25 percent of your total calories should come from foods with added sugars (soft drinks, pastries, cookies, candies, and other foods and beverages to which sugar is added during production). This maximum amount of sugars was based on evidence that people whose diets are high in added sugars have lower intakes of essential nutrients. Personally, I think that 25 percent is too high and that you should strive for 10 percent.

Dietary Fiber

Studies show that people with low-fiber diets have an increased risk of developing heart disease. There is additional evidence to suggest that more fiber in the diet helps prevent colon cancer and promotes weight control, but the findings are unconfirmed at this point.

The dietary fiber recommendations are as follows:

- **Men:** 38 grams up to age 50, and 30 grams over age 50
- **Women:** 25 grams up to age 50, and 21 grams over age 50
- **Children 1 to 3 years:** 19 grams per day
- **Children 4 to 8 years:** 25 grams per day
- **Boys 9 to 13 years:** 31 grams per day
- **Boys 14 to 18 years:** 38 grams per day
- **Girls 9 to 18 years:** 26 grams per day

Appendix E

Metric Conversion Guide

*N*ote: The recipes in this cookbook were not developed or tested using metric measures. There may be some variation in quality when converting to metric units.

Common Abbreviations

Abbreviation(s)	What It Stands For
C, c	cup
g	gram
kg	kilogram
L, l	liter
lb	pound
mL, ml	milliliter
oz	ounce
pt	pint
t, tsp	teaspoon
T, TB, Tbl, Tbsp	tablespoon

Volume

U.S. Units	Canadian Metric	Australian Metric
¼ teaspoon	1 mL	1 ml
½ teaspoon	2 mL	2 ml
1 teaspoon	5 mL	5 ml

(continued)

Volume *(continued)*

U.S. Units	Canadian Metric	Australian Metric
1 tablespoon	15 mL	20 ml
¼ cup	50 mL	60 ml
⅓ cup	75 mL	80 ml
½ cup	125 mL	125 ml
⅔ cup	150 mL	170 ml
¾ cup	175 mL	190 ml
1 cup	250 mL	250 ml
1 quart	1 liter	1 liter
1½ quarts	1.5 liters	1.5 liters
2 quarts	2 liters	2 liters
2½ quarts	2.5 liters	2.5 liters
3 quarts	3 liters	3 liters
4 quarts	4 liters	4 liters

Weight

U.S. Units	Canadian Metric	Australian Metric
1 ounce	30 grams	30 grams
2 ounces	55 grams	60 grams
3 ounces	85 grams	90 grams
4 ounces (¼ pound)	115 grams	125 grams
8 ounces (½ pound)	225 grams	225 grams
16 ounces (1 pound)	455 grams	500 grams
1 pound	455 grams	½ kilogram

Measurements

Inches	Centimeters
½	1.5
1	2.5
2	5.0
3	7.5
4	10.0
5	12.5
6	15.0
7	17.5
8	20.5
9	23.0
10	25.5
11	28.0
12	30.5
13	33.0

Temperature (Degrees)

Fahrenheit	Celsius
32	0
212	100
250	120
275	140
300	150
325	160
350	180
375	190

(continued)

Temperature (Degrees) *(continued)*

Fahrenheit	Celsius
400	200
425	220
450	230
475	240
500	260

Index

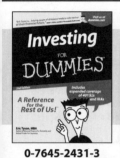
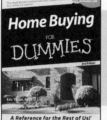
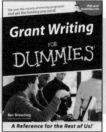
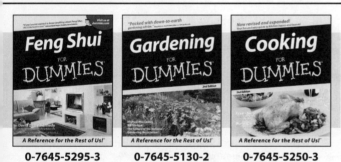
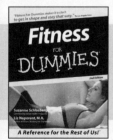
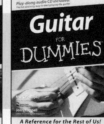
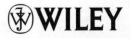

TRAVEL

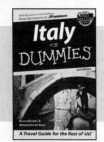

0-7645-5453-0

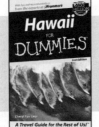

0-7645-5438-7

0-7645-5444-1

Also available:

America's National Parks For Dummies
(0-7645-6204-5)

Caribbean For Dummies
(0-7645-5445-X)

Cruise Vacations For Dummies 2003
(0-7645-5459-X)

Europe For Dummies
(0-7645-5456-5)

Ireland For Dummies
(0-7645-6199-5)

France For Dummies
(0-7645-6292-4)

Las Vegas For Dummies
(0-7645-5448-4)

London For Dummies
(0-7645-5416-6)

Mexico's Beach Resorts For Dummies
(0-7645-6262-2)

Paris For Dummies
(0-7645-5494-8)

RV Vacations For Dummies
(0-7645-5443-3)

EDUCATION & TEST PREPARATION

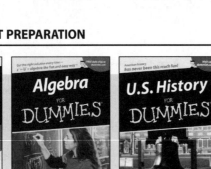

0-7645-5194-9

0-7645-5325-9

0-7645-5249-X

Also available:

The ACT For Dummies
(0-7645-5210-4)

Chemistry For Dummies
(0-7645-5430-1)

English Grammar For Dummies
(0-7645-5322-4)

French For Dummies
(0-7645-5193-0)

GMAT For Dummies
(0-7645-5251-1)

Inglés Para Dummies
(0-7645-5427-1)

Italian For Dummies
(0-7645-5196-5)

Research Papers For Dummies
(0-7645-5426-3)

SAT I For Dummies
(0-7645-5472-7)

U.S. History For Dummies
(0-7645-5249-X)

World History For Dummies
(0-7645-5242-2)

HEALTH, SELF-HELP & SPIRITUALITY

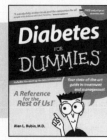

0-7645-5154-X

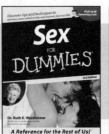

0-7645-5302-X

0-7645-5418-2

Also available:

The Bible For Dummies
(0-7645-5296-1)

Controlling Cholesterol For Dummies
(0-7645-5440-9)

Dating For Dummies
(0-7645-5072-1)

Dieting For Dummies
(0-7645-5126-4)

High Blood Pressure For Dummies
(0-7645-5424-7)

Judaism For Dummies
(0-7645-5299-6)

Menopause For Dummies
(0-7645-5458-1)

Nutrition For Dummies
(0-7645-5180-9)

Potty Training For Dummies
(0-7645-5417-4)

Pregnancy For Dummies
(0-7645-5074-8)

Rekindling Romance For Dummies
(0-7645-5303-8)

Religion For Dummies
(0-7645-5264-3)

FOR DUMMIES®

Plain-English solutions for everyday challenges

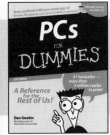
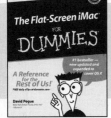
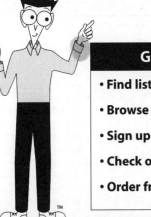
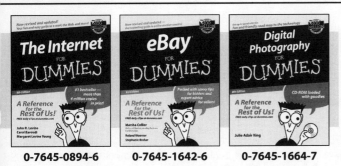

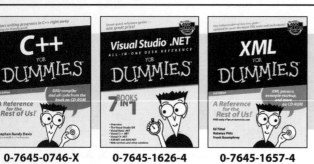

FOR DUMMIES

Helping you expand your horizons and realize your potential

GRAPHICS & WEB SITE DEVELOPMENT

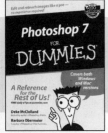

Photoshop 7 FOR DUMMIES

A Reference for the Rest of Us!

Deke McClelland
Barbara Obermeier

0-7645-1651-5

Creating Web Pages FOR DUMMIES

A Reference for the Rest of Us!

Bud Smith
Arthur Bebak

0-7645-1643-4

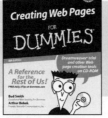

Macromedia Flash MX FOR DUMMIES

A Reference for the Rest of Us!

Gurdy Leete
Ellen Finkelstein

0-7645-0895-4

Also available:

Adobe Acrobat 5 PDF For Dummies
(0-7645-1652-3)

ASP.NET For Dummies
(0-7645-0866-0)

ColdFusion MX For Dummies
(0-7645-1672-8)

Dreamweaver MX For Dummies
(0-7645-1630-2)

FrontPage 2002 For Dummies
(0-7645-0821-0)

HTML 4 For Dummies
(0-7645-0723-0)

Illustrator 10 For Dummies
(0-7645-3636-2)

PowerPoint 2002 For Dummies
(0-7645-0817-2)

Web Design For Dummies
(0-7645-0823-7)

PROGRAMMING & DATABASES

C++ FOR DUMMIES

A Reference for the Rest of Us!

Stephen Randy Davis

0-7645-0746-X

Visual Studio .NET ALL-IN-ONE DESK REFERENCE FOR DUMMIES

7 BOOKS IN 1

0-7645-1626-4

XML FOR DUMMIES

A Reference for the Rest of Us!

Ed Tittel
Natanya Pitts
Frank Boumphrey

0-7645-1657-4

Also available:

Access 2002 For Dummies
(0-7645-0818-0)

Beginning Programming For Dummies
(0-7645-0835-0)

Crystal Reports 9 For Dummies
(0-7645-1641-8)

Java & XML For Dummies
(0-7645-1658-2)

Java 2 For Dummies
(0-7645-0765-6)

JavaScript For Dummies
(0-7645-0633-1)

Oracle9i For Dummies
(0-7645-0880-6)

Perl For Dummies
(0-7645-0776-1)

PHP and MySQL For Dummies
(0-7645-1650-7)

SQL For Dummies
(0-7645-0737-0)

Visual Basic .NET For Dummies
(0-7645-0867-9)

LINUX, NETWORKING & CERTIFICATION

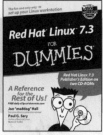

Red Hat Linux 7.3 FOR DUMMIES

A Reference for the Rest of Us!

Jon "maddog" Hall
Paul G. Sery

0-7645-1545-4

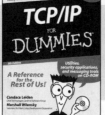

TCP/IP FOR DUMMIES

A Reference for the Rest of Us!

Candace Leiden
Marshall Wilensky

0-7645-1760-0

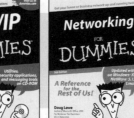

Networking FOR DUMMIES

A Reference for the Rest of Us!

Doug Lowe

0-7645-0772-9

Also available:

A+ Certification For Dummies
(0-7645-0812-1)

CCNP All-in-One Certification For Dummies
(0-7645-1648-5)

Cisco Networking For Dummies
(0-7645-1668-X)

CISSP For Dummies
(0-7645-1670-1)

CIW Foundations For Dummies
(0-7645-1635-3)

Firewalls For Dummies
(0-7645-0884-9)

Home Networking For Dummies
(0-7645-0857-1)

Red Hat Linux All-in-One Desk Reference For Dummies
(0-7645-2442-9)

UNIX For Dummies
(0-7645-0419-3)

Available wherever books are sold.
Go to www.dummies.com or call 1-877-762-2974 to order direct

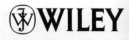

WILEY